Speech Therapy Aphasia Rehabilitation
STAR
Workbook

Amanda Anderson M.S. CCC-SLP

About the Author:

Amanda Anderson is a Speech-Language Pathologist and has worked in a combination of assisted living, skilled nursing, outpatient, and acute care settings with adults. She specializes in stroke rehabilitation in both speech, language and swallowing disorders. She graduated with honors from Davidson College in Davidson, North Carolina. She received her Master's Degree in Speech-Language Pathology from the University of Hawaii. She holds her certificate of clinical competence from the American Speech-Language-Hearing association in Speech-Language Pathology. She has published one other work with McFarland as an editor for her late grandfather Louis Lauria's war memoir, *Running Wire on the Front Lines*. She created this workbook for her patients to use at home to continue therapy after their Medicare therapy benefits were unable to cover further rehabilitation.

Dedication:
Dedicated to Carolee Gramaglia whose motivation
and tenacity has been a true inspiration.

Table of Contents

Introduction	1
Workbook Instructions for Family Members	2
Carrier Phrases	5
Functional Picture Naming	34
Rote Naming	84
Convergent Naming	86
Divergent Naming	90
Melodic Intonation Exercises	97
Functional Writing Exercises	103
Describing Functions of Objects	108
"Wh" Questions	110
Reading Exercises	121
Describing Picture Scenes	124
Conversation Exercises	144

Take Action!

I wrote this book for several of my patients because their Medicare part B benefits no longer covered speech therapy. All too often, individuals who have a stroke resulting in aphasia also need physical therapy. Currently, there is a therapy cap of $1,900 for both speech-language pathology and physical therapy combined. Rarely is this enough to support patients through a full physical and language recovery.

Please take action! Contact your representatives and let them know how the therapy caps have negatively impacted you. The American Speech-Language and Hearing Association has an easy form to email to your members of Congress. Visit their website asha.org and under the advocacy tab you will find the take action section to contact Congress to repeal the medicare part B caps. Currently, the link to the form is:

http://takeaction.asha.org/asha2/issues/alert/?alertid=62421566

Introduction

This workbook was created for people with aphasia to use with their speech therapist or with a caregiver at home in order to improve their expressive language. Aphasia is not a progressive disease. There is a strong potential for recovery of language skills with therapy, motivation, and a lot of support. Unfortunately, insurance often doesn't cover speech therapy long enough to regain prior communication levels. This workbook is meant to serve as a supplement to therapy or to guide family through therapy to improve their loved one's expressive language.

The language center of the brain (Broca's area) is typically in the left hemisphere. Aphasia is a result of damage to this area of the brain from a stroke either caused by lack of oxygen (ischemic stroke) or bleeding in the brain (hemorrhagic stroke). After a stroke resulting in aphasia, the words and knowledge haven't been forgotten, the neurological pathways have just been damaged. Think of a stroke as a road block in the brain. The words are still there but the pathways to retrieve them have been damaged.

Speech therapy works by recruiting undamaged areas of the brain to help retrieve appropriate words during expressive communication. The goal of speech therapy is to use other "roads" to retrieve the words. Music, rhythm, gestures, adjectives and adverbs help the brain find other routes to communicate. A person with aphasia can use gestures, writing, sounds, music, rhythm and other descriptive terms to recruit other areas of the brain to improve expressive language.

The brain is capable of creating new neurological pathways to "detour" around damaged areas. The key to successful aphasia speech therapy is to build these new neurological pathways. Speech therapy helps create these new neurological pathways and the exercises in this workbook are helpful tools to improve communication skills after a stroke. Because Aphasia is not a memory disorder, using exercises with well know phrases, songs and sayings help utilize memory to increase the brain's ability to form "detours" around the damaged areas to improve expressive language. Frequent practice of these exercises increases the formation of new neurological pathways to improve communication.

Try to use the exercises from this workbook daily. Repetition of successful language activities helps increase communication. The most important thing for a family member or caregiver to remember is that true aphasia does not damage your loved one's cognitive abilities. Remind your loved one that you understand they know the answer and they are just having difficulty expressing it. The answers to the questions in the workbook are designed to be easy and they are not meant to question the patient's intelligence but rather to improve their ability to retrieve words. As you move through this workbook it is important to know that frustration is a natural part of aphasia therapy. Frustration can exacerbate word finding difficulties and it is especially important to learn to relax and not let frustration become a form of language blockage. If you get frustrated, take a break.

How To Use This Workbook

Speech-Language Pathologists

As you are aware, insurance often doesn't cover speech therapy long enough to support a patient with aphasia through a full recovery. I wrote this book for my patients to use at home with a partner to increase carryover of expressive language skills with homework exercises and to continue use after they were discharged from therapy. This workbook can also be utilized throughout therapy to achieve multiple goals. I especially wanted to include full color photographs for both functional naming and descriptive language which is an important aspect of therapy for a person with aphasia. This workbook includes sections appropriate for patients with severe expressive aphasia (rote naming, carrier phrases, and functional naming) as well as more advanced exercises (function of objects, divergent naming, describing photographs, conversation topics and functional writing exercises).

For Family and Caregivers

This workbook is also designed to be used at home by the patient individually or with the help of a family member. Everyone has experienced the feeling of having a word on the "tip of their tongue". Keep in mind, somebody with aphasia has this experience constantly and struggles to find the words they want to say even though they know what they want to say. The exercises are structured by difficulty level and each exercise is an opportunity to improve word retrieval skills.

Carrier Phrases make up the first section of the book. These exercises help increase word retrieval by utilizing memory and lead in cues to help produce the desired word. Initially, read the phrase to your partner with aphasia and pause for them to fill in the blank. If your partner is unable to say the desired word, try making the first sound of the word. This is called a phonemic cue. For example: read "An apple a day keeps the doctor" and then make the "a" sound for away. If they still have difficulty, have them repeat the completed phrase after you. Once the phrases become easier, have your partner read the phrase aloud themselves and complete it.

Functional Picture Naming: The objective here is for the person with aphasia to name the item in the photograph. If they have trouble, use the carrier phrases below each picture. The questions below each photo are designed to help form new pathways to increase expressive language. Finding other ways to describe an item by function, or using a gesture, helps work around the area of the brain that was damaged. If your partner is unable to name or answer any of the questions about the photo, write the name of the picture on an index card and place it below the picture. Have them read it with the picture. Practice reading the words with the pictures and gradually remove the written cue once they are able to read the name with the photograph on a consistent basis. Also, try having your partner write the name of the picture. Depending on the type of stroke, writing can be just as difficult as speaking or it can be unaffected and a perfect mode of communication to help facilitate speech.

Rote Naming: Contains exercises to use with people with severe expressive aphasia. Counting and the alphabet are automatic parts of language that we have memorized. Using rhythm and music can help increase accuracy with these exercises. Practice saying them together and gradually back down and let your partner read them on their own and then say them by heart.

Convergent Naming: These are descriptions of items. Read a few of the sentences and see if your partner can guess what is being described. If they are not able to say the item, read the carrier phrase at the end. If they still can't say the item, try adding some descriptions of your own and see if your partner can make a gesture pretending they are using the item.

Divergent Naming: This section focuses on categories. Broad categories typically are the most challenging. The first exercises help break down broad categories into subcategories. Encourage the use of visualization to help think of items in categories. For example, if the category is vegetables, picture a salad or the produce section of the grocery store.

Melodic Intonation: Music Therapy is an excellent way to utilize undamaged areas of the brain to help increase expressive language. Try singing the songs in the workbook together. Also, play your partner's favorite songs and try singing along to them. Use songs they know very well. It should be a memory and singing exercises instead of a reading exercise.

Functional Writing Exercises: Use these forms to practice writing. Depending on the type of stroke, writing can be just as difficult as speaking and word finding difficulties can also occur with writing. Try filling out a form as an example for your partner and have them practice copying their personal information onto a new blank copy of the form.

Function of Items: This is a higher level exercise to focus on describing using action words, adjectives, and gestures. Any information your partner can express is encouraging. Try to cue the person with aphasia by asking them what they do with each item or have them pretend they are using the item.

"Wh" Questions: This is also a higher level exercise. Encourage descriptions of the answer instead of just focusing on a name. Try to read your partner's expressions. After working together for awhile, you should be able to tell when they know the answer. If a question is too difficult, skip it and come back to it later. Too much frustration caused by working on questions that are difficult can be detrimental to therapy. It is more productive to have a lot of success with easy questions as long as you are practicing frequently and continue to form new neurological connections. The goal is to have your partner decrease the level of cues they need to say the correct answer in each exercise.

Reading Exercises: Depending on the type of stroke, your loved one may have difficulty reading. Aphasia may impact their ability to retrieve the word despite having the written word in front of them. Apraxia, a disorder in coordinating and initiating the muscle movements required to speak, could also be a factor here. Try reading the phrases aloud with your partner. Pace out each word slowly and point to it as you go. It is common for somebody with aphasia to skip words because they are reading the words much faster than they are able to say them aloud. Once your partner is able to read the phrases and sentences in the workbook, practice reading from newspapers or from books. The fluency developed while reading aloud will help with recovery of spontaneous speech.

Describing Photographs: The goal of this exercise is to have your partner give as much detail about each photo as possible. Naming isn't the goal here. Try giving them the book without knowing the picture they are looking at. Encourage them to describe colors, people, time of year, location etc. Use the pictures to start conversations about places and personal experiences.

Conversation Starters: The first portion contains structured conversations. Ask your partner the question. Once they answer, have them ask you the same question back. Continue to practice these conversation sets multiple times. Initiating conversation and asking questions can be extremely challenging for somebody with aphasia. The next set of questions in this section are designed to start conversations. Use them together or have your loved one practice with another family member or friend. Some of the questions are meant to be controversial to start a conversation. You know your partner best, so select questions you think they would enjoy talking about.

Speech therapy for aphasia can be a long process. Remember that progress does happen. Patient motivation is a key factor for recovery. Warm up with activities from the book that are easy. Move on to more difficult sections but only for 10 to 15 minutes if they are frustrating for your partner. Cool down with activities that are easier. Frequent success and a lot of practice is the key to progress. Having the determination to work together to improve expressive language skills is a huge step in the right direction.

Carrier Phrases

Level 1: Read the phrase aloud and pause to let your partner finish the phrase.
Level 2: Have your partner read the sentence aloud and complete it.
Level 3. Patient should read the sentence aloud and say and write in the answer.

1. An apple a day keeps the doctor _____.

2. His bark is worse than his _____.

3. Three little kittens have lost their _____.

4. Rubber ducky you're the one. You make bath time so much _____.

5. Head and shoulders, knees and _____.

6. One hand washes the _____.

7. Put your pants on one leg at a _____.

8. I'm a monkey's _____.

9. A penny saved is a penny _____.

10. Absence makes the heart grow _____.

11. Everything happens for a _____.

12. The pen is mightier than the _____.

13. Good things come to those who _____.

14. The meek shall inherit the _____.

15. If its not one thing it's _____.

Carrier Phrases

Common Sayings:

1. Between a rock and a hard _____.

2. Cut off your nose to spite your _____.

3. Like looking for a needle in a _____.

4. Barking up the wrong _____.

5. It's always in the last place you _____.

6. It is what it _____.

7. Time to hit the ground _____.

8. With all due _____.

9. To make a long story _____.

10. Let's not re-invent the _____.

11. Kill two birds with one _____.

12. Why did the chicken cross the _____?

13. Every cloud has a silver _____.

14. Takes one to know _____.

15. Don't take this the wrong _____.

Carrier Phrases

Common Sayings:

1. Better late than _____.

2. Skeletons in your _____.

3. Don't judge a book by its _____.

4. If at first you don't succeed, try, try_____.

5. Two heads are better than _____.

6. If you want something done right, do it _____.

7. No rest for the _____.

8. Swallowed it, hook, line and _____.

9. The bigger they are, the harder they _____.

10. Its not rocket _____.

11. The pot calling the kettle _____.

12. The goose that lays the golden _____.

13. Just made it by the skin of my _____.

14. Cleanliness is next to _____.

15. Eat your heart _____.

Carrier Phrases

Common Sayings:

1. A bird in the hand is worth two in the _____.

2. A house divided against itself cannot _____.

3. A drop in the _____.

4. A labor of _____.

5. A leopard cannot change its _____.

6. A man after my own _____.

7. Am I my brother's _____?

8. An eye for an eye, a tooth for a _____.

9. Ashes to ashes, dust to _____.

10. Eat drink and be _____.

11. He who lives by the sword dies by the _____.

12. It is better to give than to _____.

13. Let he who is without sin cast the first _____.

14. Living off the fat of the _____.

15. Stop putting words in my _____.

Carrier Phrases

Common Sayings:

1. Spare the rod and spoil the _____.

2. The apple of my _____.

3. The blind leading the _____.

4. I'll follow you to the ends of the _____.

5. The love of money is the root of all _____.

6. The salt of the _____.

7. The spirit is willing but the flesh is _____.

8. Read the writing on the _____.

9. You reap what you _____.

10. A plague on both your _____.

11. As pure as the driven _____.

12. Eaten out of house and _____.

13. Wear my heart upon my _____.

14. The game is _____.

15. Led me on a wild goose _____.

Carrier Phrases

Common Sayings:

1. A chain is only as strong as its weakest _____.

2. A dog is a man's best _____.

3. A fool and his money are soon _____.

4. A little knowledge is a dangerous _____.

5. A picture is worth a thousand _____.

6. A place for everything and everything in its _____.

7. A good man is hard to _____.

8. A rolling stone gathers no _____.

9. A stitch in time saves _____.

10. A watched pot never _____.

11. A woman's work is never _____.

12. Actions speak louder than _____.

13. All good things must come to an _____.

14. All roads lead to _____.

15. All work and no play makes Jack a dull _____.

Carrier Phrases

Common Sayings:

1. All you need is _____.

2. All's fair in love and _____.

3. All's well that ends _____.

4. An army marches on its _____.

5. Another day another _____.

6. April showers bring May _____.

7. As thick as _____.

8. Beauty is in the eye of the _____.

9. Behind every great man there's a great _____.

10. Better safe than _____.

11. Better to have loved and lost than never to have loved _____.

12. Birds of a feather flock _____.

13. Boys will be _____.

14. Business before _____.

15. Cheaters never _____.

Carrier Phrases

Common Sayings:

1. Children should be seen and not _____.

2. Clothes make the _____.

3. Cold hands, warm _____.

4. Count your _____.

5. Don't count your chickens before they _____.

6. Crime doesn't _____.

7. Do as I say not as I _____.

8. Do unto others as you would have them do unto _____.

9. Don't bite the hand that feeds _____.

10. Don't change horses mid _____.

11. We will cross that bridge when we come _____.

12. Don't put all your eggs in one _____.

13. Don't rock the _____.

14. Don't throw the baby out with the _____.

15. Early to bed early to _____.

Carrier Phrases

Common Sayings:

1. Easy come easy _____.

2. Enough is _____!

3. Every dog has his _____.

4. First come first _____.

5. Fight fire with _____.

6. Fish and guests smell after three _____.

7. Forgive and _____.

8. Give credit where credit is _____.

9. God helps those who help _____.

10. Great minds think _____.

11. Haste makes _____.

12. Home is where the _____ is.

13. Honesty is the best _____.

14. If it ain't broke, don't fix _____.

15. It ain't over until the fat lady _____.

Carrier Phrases

Common Sayings:

1. If the shoe fits _____.

2. If you can't beat em, join _____.

3. If you can't stand the heat, get out of the _____.

4. It takes two to _____.

5. No use crying over spilt _____.

6. The squeaky wheel gets the _____.

7. Keep your chin _____.

8. Laugh and the world laughs with _____.

9. Laughter is the best _____.

10. Less is _____.

11. Let bygones be _____.

12. Let sleeping dogs _____.

13. Let the punishment fit the _____.

14. Let well enough _____.

15. Life is like a box of _____.

Carrier Phrases

Common Sayings:

1. Lightning never strikes twice in the same _____.

2. Like father like _____.

3. Let sleeping dogs _____.

4. Look before you _____.

5. Love is all you _____.

6. Love makes the world go _____.

7. I'm going to make an offer he can't _____.

8. March: goes in like a lion and out like a _____.

9. Life is a bowl of _____.

10. Money doesn't grow on _____.

11. Never put off until tomorrow what you can do _____.

12. Nothing ventured nothing _____.

13. Patience is a _____.

14. People who live in glass houses shouldn't throw _____.

15. Practice makes _____.

Carrier Phrases

Common Sayings:

1. Put your best foot _____.

2. The apple never falls too far from the _____.

3. The best defence is a good _____.

4. The best things in life are _____.

5. Only the good die _____.

6. The more the _____.

7. The proof is in the _____.

8. The way to a man's heart is through his _____.

9. Time flies when you are having _____.

10. Waste not want _____.

11. What goes up must come _____.

12. You are what you _____.

13. Youth is wasted on the _____.

14. Two wrongs don't make a _____.

15. You can't make an omelet without breaking a few _____.

Carrier Phrases

Logical Answers:

1. I'm so sleepy, I should go to _____.

2. It's a beautiful summer day. I'm going to swim in the _____.

3. I'd like to order a bacon, lettuce and _____ sandwich.

4. The best things in life are _____.

5. Airport security always has such long _____.

6. I better go online and check my _____.

7. In the morning, to wake up I have to have a cup of _____.

8. I'm going to the beach, can't forget a bucket and _____.

9. I'm going to bake some chocolate chip _____.

10. Looks like rain today so don't forget to bring an _____.

11. As a thank you they sent her a large fruit _____.

12. After driving 2,500 miles, I should get an oil _____.

13. Oh no, Scrappy looks hungry, I need to go buy some dog _____.

14. Please put this screwdriver away in my tool _____.

15. On Saturday mornings, I love to shop at garage _____.

Carrier Phrases

Logical Answers:

1. I'm going to buy an Angel Fish for my fish _____.

2. It is very sunny so I am wearing sun_____.

3. Let's go see the elephants and gorillas at the city _____.

4. Blow out the candles on your birthday _____.

5. I have to go to the ATM and get some _____.

6. I'm going to have steak and a baked _____.

7. They need to cut down that tree with a chain_____.

8. Bring over that topsoil in the wheel_____.

9. The kids at the park played base_____.

10. I'm not sure if it is easier to take the bus or the sub_____.

11. I'm worried that a motorcycle isn't very _____.

12. We went to Florida to watch the space shuttle _____.

13. S'mores have graham crackers, marshmallows and _____.

14. This weekend I'm going to go horseback _____.

15. I'd like to change the TV channel. Please hand me the _____.

Carrier Phrases

Logical Answers:

1. The floor is so dirty, I need to use the vacuum _____.

2. I have to put this letter in the mail _____.

3. "Ring" "Ring" Please answer the _____.

4. For breakfast, I would like bacon and _____.

5. Wash your hands with soap and _____.

6. It's way too loud to sleep. I need to put in ear _____.

7. Please help me! I'm in the bathroom and we are out of toilet _____.

8. My nails are uneven. I need to use a nail _____.

9. We are low on food. It is time to go grocery _____.

10. Are we going to have a party on Super Bowl _____?

11. In the morning, I take my multi - _____.

12. I'd like something different tonight. Let's eat out at a _____.

13. A woman can never have too many pairs of _____.

14. Today is our anniversary. 40 years ago we got _____.

15. Oh no, I dropped that. Could you please pick it _____?

Carrier Phrases

Song Titles from the 70s

1. Johnny Nash: "I Can See Clearly _____"

2. Don McLean: "American _____"

3. ABBA: "Dancing _____"

4. Gloria Gaynor: "I Will _____"

5. The Cars: "Just What I _____"

6. Cheap Trick: "I Want You to Want _____"

7. Bee Gees: "Stayin' _____"

8. Led Zeppelin: "Stairway to _____"

9. John Denver: "Thank God I'm a Country _____"

10. Carly Simon: "Your so _____"

11. Steely Dan: "Reelin in the _____"

12. Roberta Flack: "Killing Me _____"

13. James Taylor: "Fire and _____"

14. The Eagles: "One of these _____"

15. Pink Floyd: "Wish you were _____"

Carrier Phrases

60s Song Titles:

1. You Are So Beautiful To _____.

2. I Wanna Hold Your _____.

3. Duke of _____.

4. With a Little Help From My _____.

5. Bad Moon _____.

6. Blow'in in the _____.

7. Build Me Up _____.

8. Sugar Pie Honey _____.

9. You Make Me Feel Like a Natural _____.

10. Brown Eyed _____.

11. Sittin On The Dock of the _____.

12. Jumpin' Jack _____.

13. You Can't Always Get What You _____.

14. When a Man Loves a _____.

15. Ain't too Proud to _____.

Carrier Phrases

50s Song Titles:

1. Rock Around the _____.

2. Wake Up Little _____.

3. Yakety _____.

4. Little Bitty Pretty _____.

5. Whole lot of Shakin' Going _____.

6. Blue Suede _____.

7. In the Still of the _____.

8. Heartbreak _____.

9. One Eyed, One Horned, Flying Purple People _____.

10. Why do Fools Fall in _____.

11. Bridge Over Troubled _____.

12. I Walk the _____.

13. How much is that Doggie in the _____?

14. Great Balls of _____.

15. You ain't Nothing but a Hound _____.

Carrier Phrases

Patriotic Song Titles:

1. Yankee _____.

2. God Bless _____.

3. Born in the _____.

4. Star Spangled _____.

5. This Land is Your _____.

6. Battle Hymn of the _____.

7. When Johnny Comes Marching _____.

8. Stars and Stripes _____.

9. My Country Tis of _____.

10. America the _____.

Carrier Phrases

Holiday Songs:

1. I'm Dreaming of a White _____.

2. Rudolf the Red Nose _____.

3. Frosty the _____.

4. Jingle _____.

5. I'll be Home for _____.

6. Silent _____.

7. Let it _____.

8. Away in a _____.

9. Jolly Old Saint _____.

10. O Little Town of _____.

11. Up on the _____.

12. Oh Christmas _____.

13. Deck the _____.

14. Santa Claus is Coming to _____.

15. O Come all Ye _____.

Carrier Phrases

Movie Titles:

1. The Sound of _____.

2. Star _____.

3. Born on the 4th of _____.

4. Snow White and the Seven _____.

5. Gone with the _____.

6. Blazing _____.

7. Around the World in 80 _____.

8. The Lord of the _____.

9. My Fair _____.

10. Jurassic _____.

11. It's a Wonderful _____.

12. Alice in _____.

13. The Wizard of _____.

14. Forrest _____.

15. My Big Fat Greek _____.

Carrier Phrases

Popular TV Shows:

1. Everybody Loves _____.

2. All in the _____.

3. The Brady _____.

4. The Days of Our _____.

5. As the World _____.

6. The Cosby _____.

7. I Love _____.

8. The Late Show with David _____.

9. Father Knows _____.

10. The Dick Van _____.

11. The Twilight _____.

12. The X-_____.

13. The Oprah _____.

14. Hawaii _____

15. Law & _____.

Carrier Phrases

Sports Teams: Baseball

1. Baltimore _____.

2. Boston Red _____.

3. Chicago White _____.

4. Cleveland _____.

5. Detroit _____.

6. Atlanta _____.

7. New York _____.

8. Philadelphia _____.

9. St. Louis _____.

10. San Francisco _____.

Carrier Phrases

Sports Teams: Football

1. Pittsburgh _____.

2. Baltimore _____.

3. Cleveland _____.

4. Green Bay _____.

5. Carolina _____.

6. Chicago _____.

7. Dallas _____.

8. San Francisco _____.

9. Washington _____.

10. Philadelphia_____.

11. New York _____.

12. Denver_____.

13. Oakland _____.

14. Miami _____.

15. New England _____.

Carrier Phrases

Meals and Dishes

1. Chicken Cordon _____.

2. Shepard's _____.

3. Spaghetti and _____.

4. Caesar _____.

5. Fettuccine _____.

6. Grilled Rib- Eye _____.

7. Macaroni and _____.

8. Sweet and Sour _____.

9. French _____.

10. Pineapple upside down _____.

11. Peanut Butter and _____.

12. Mashed _____.

13. Oysters on the half _____.

14. Cream of Mushroom _____.

15. Loaded Baked _____.

Carrier Phrases

Name the State that goes with each city:

1. Newark, _____

2. Philadelphia, _____.

3. Boston, _____.

4. New Haven, _____.

5. Chicago, _____.

6. Tampa, _____.

7. Atlanta, _____.

8. Pittsburgh, _____.

9. Cleveland, _____.

10. New Orleans, _____.

11. New York, _____.

12. San Francisco, _____.

13. Phoenix, _____.

14. Las Vegas, _____.

15. Los Angeles, _____.

Carrier Phrases

Nursery Rhymes

1. Hickory, Dickory, Dock the mouse went up the _____.

2. Pat-a-Cake Pat-a-Cake, baker's man bake me a cake as fast as you _____.

3. Rub-a-dub-dub, three men in a _____.

4. This little piggy went to _____.

5. Peter, Peter, pumpkin _____.

6. Jack be nimble, Jack be quick, Jack jump over the _____.

7. Georgie Porgie, pudding pie, kissed the girls and made them _____.

8. Jack and Jill went up the _____.

9. Little Miss Muffet sat on a _____.

10. Humpty Dumpty sat on a wall. Humpty Dumpty had a great _____.

11. All around the mulberry bush, the monkey chased the _____.

12. London Bridge is falling _____.

13. Row, row, row you boat, gently down the _____.

14. Old King Cole was a merry old _____.

15. There was an old woman who lived in a _____.

Carrier Phrases

Advertisements:

1. Pringles: "Once you pop, you can't _____."

2. "Beef it's what's for _____."

3. "This is your brain. This is your brain on _____."

4. "I've fallen and I can't get _____."

5. "Pardon me but do you have any Grey _____?"

6. "The best part of waking up is Folgers in your _____."

7. "Rice-A-Roni, the San Francisco _____."

8. "Gimme a Break. Break me off a piece of that Kit Kat _____."

9. "A diamond is _____."

10. M&Ms "melt in your mouth, not in your _____."

11. "Wheaties the breakfast of _____."

12. Timex: "Takes a licking and keeps on _____."

13. Nike: "Just do _____."

14. "Nobody better lay a finger on my _____."

15. American Express: "Don't leave home without _____."

Carrier Phrases

Movie Quotes:

Finish the quote and name the movie it is from.

1. "Frankly, my dear, I don't give a _____."

2. "I'm going to make him an offer he can't _____."

3. "Here's looking at you_____."

4. "Toto, I've got a feeling we're not in Kansas _____."

5. "Go ahead, make my _____."

6. " Louis, I think this is the beginning of a beautiful _____."

7. "Elementary my dear _____."

8. "I'm mad as hell, and I'm not going to take it _____!"

9. "Every time a bell rings an angel gets his _____."

10. "Why don't you come up sometime and see _____."

11. "I'll have what she's _____."

12. "Ask yourself one question: 'Do I feel lucky?" Well do ya _____"

13. "Mrs. Robinson, you're trying to _____ me."

14. "May the force be with _____."

15. "Say 'hello' to my little _____."

Naming Functional Objects

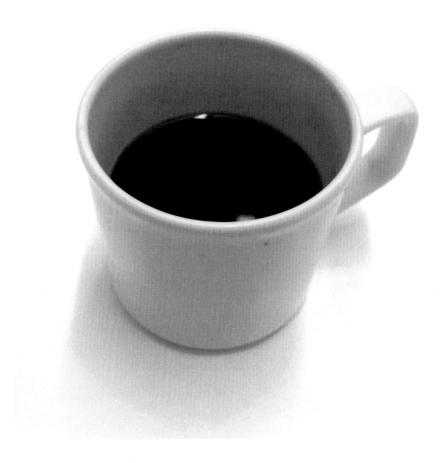

1. Pour some coffee in my _____.

2. What do you use it for?

3. Who uses it?

4. Where could you find it?

5. Use a gesture pretending to use it.

Naming Functional Objects

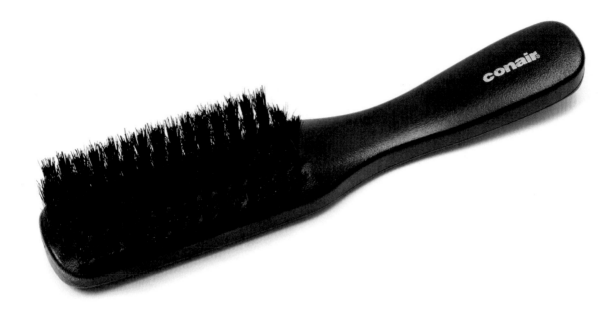

ii

1. My hair is a mess. I need to use my hair _____.

2. How do you use it?

3. When do you use it?

4. Where would you find one?

5. Pretend to use one.

Naming Functional Objects

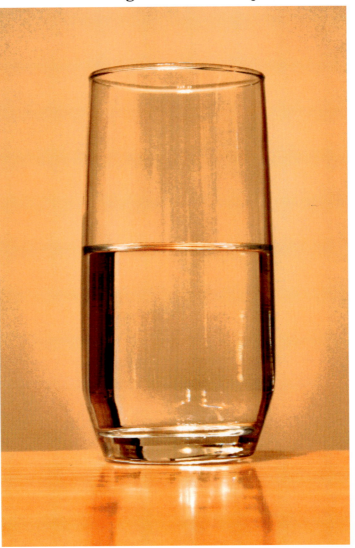

iii

1. I'm thirsty, I need a glass of _____.

2. What do you do with it?

3. Where do you find it?

4. When do you use it?

5. Show a gesture of yourself drinking it.

Naming Functional Objects

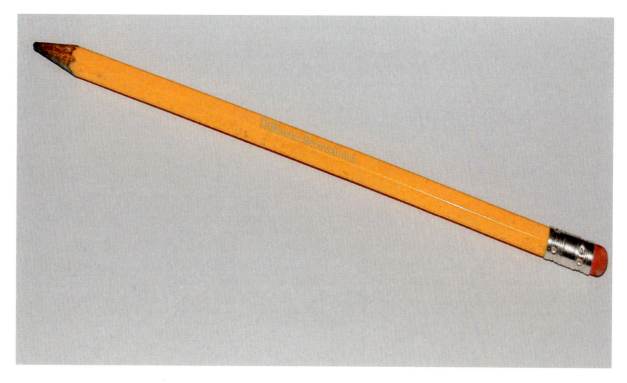

iv

1. I'll write my name, if I can borrow your _____.

2. What is it used for?

3. Where do you keep it?

4. How do you use it?

5. Pretend to write with one.

Naming Functional Objects

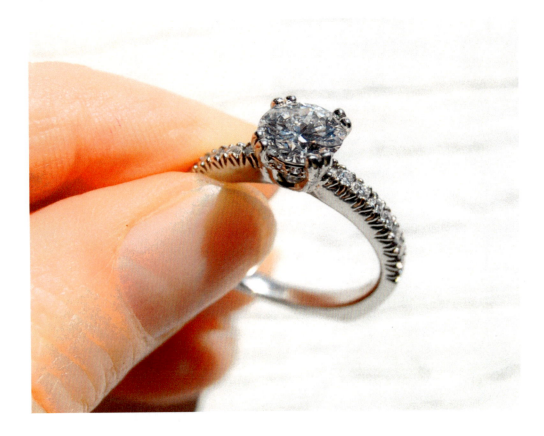

v

1. He gave her a beautiful diamond _____.

2. Who wears it?

3. Where do you wear it?

4. When do you wear one?

5. Show a gesture of putting one on.

Naming Functional Objects

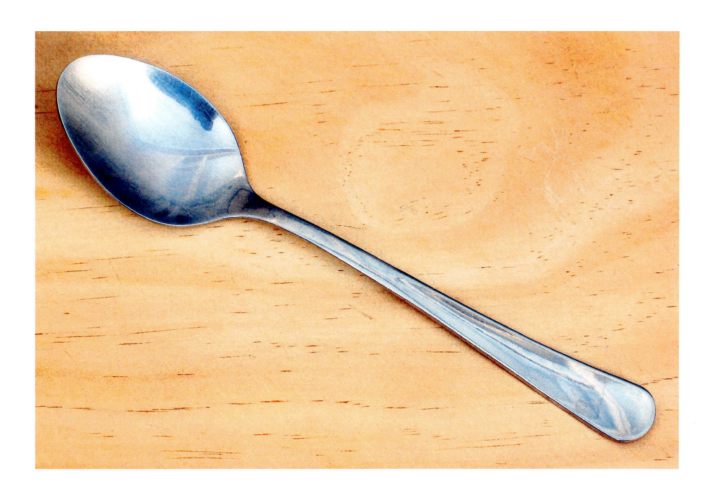

vi

1. I eat yogurt with a _____.

2. What do you do with it?

3. Where would you find one?

4. When do you use it?

5. Show a gesture of yourself using one.

Naming Functional Objects

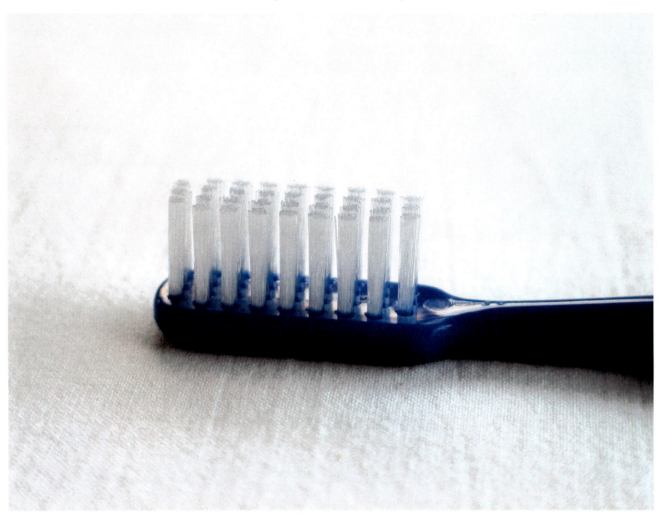

vii

1. I put toothpaste on my _____.

2. When do you use it?

3. Who uses it?

4. How do you use it?

5. Show a gesture pretending to use it.

Naming Functional Objects

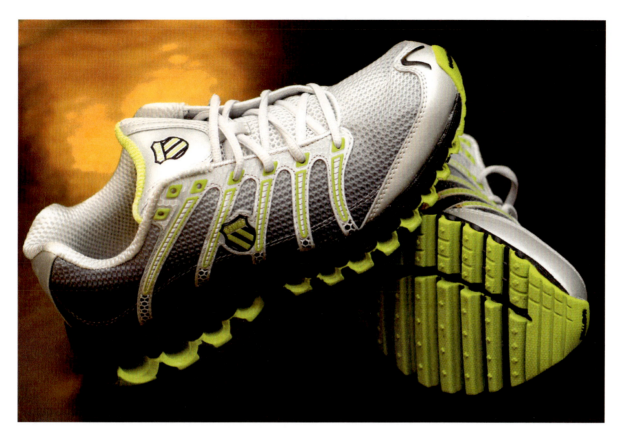

viii

1. I need to tie my _____.

2. Where do you wear them?

3. When do you wear them?

4. Who wears them?

5. Show a gesture pretending to put one on.

Naming Functional Objects

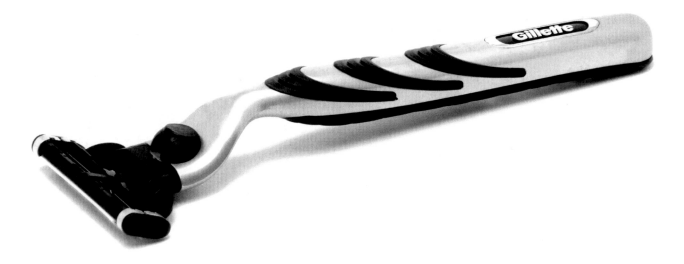

1. He shaved his beard with a _____.

2. What do you use it for?

3. When do you use it?

4. Who uses it?

5. Pretend you are using one.

Naming Functional Objects

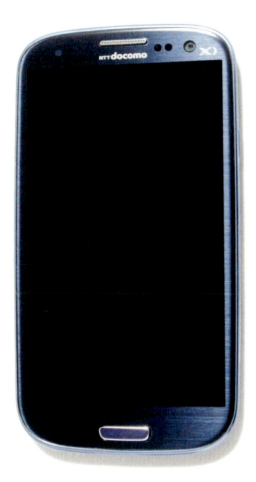

x

1. I need to make a call on my cell _____.

2. What do you do with it?

3. Where can you use it?

4. When should you never use it?

5. Pretend to talk on one.

Naming Functional Objects

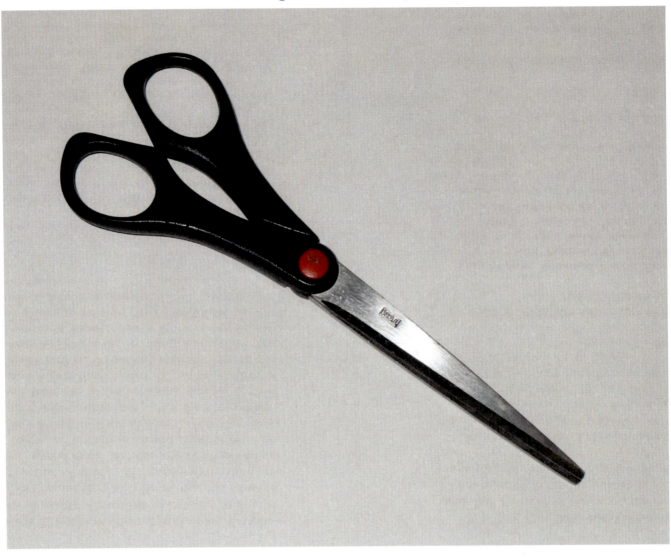

xi

1. I'll cut the wrapping paper with a pair of _____.

2. What do you do with them?

3. Where can you find them?

4. How do you use them?

5. Pretend to use them.

Naming Functional Objects

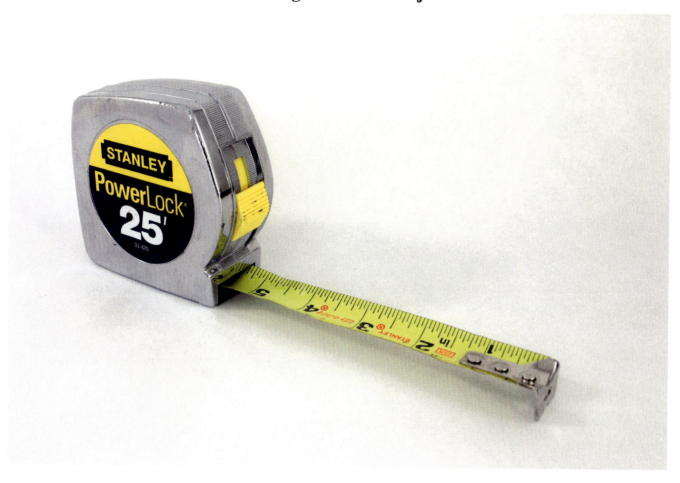

1. Get the dimensions by using a tape _____.

2. How do you use it?

3. What do you use it for?

4. Who uses it?

5. Pretend to use one.

Naming Functional Objects

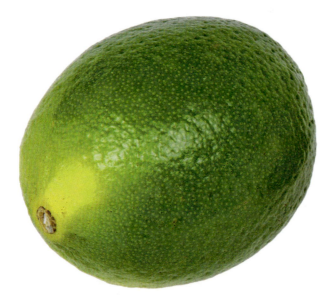
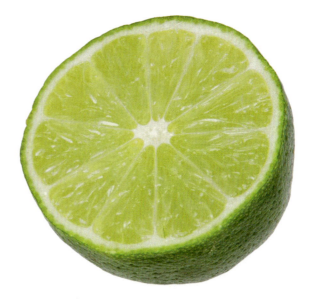

xiii

1. I'd like a Corona with a wedge of _____.

2. What colour is it?

3. Where would you find one?

4. When would you have one?

5. Pretend you tasted it.

Naming Functional Objects

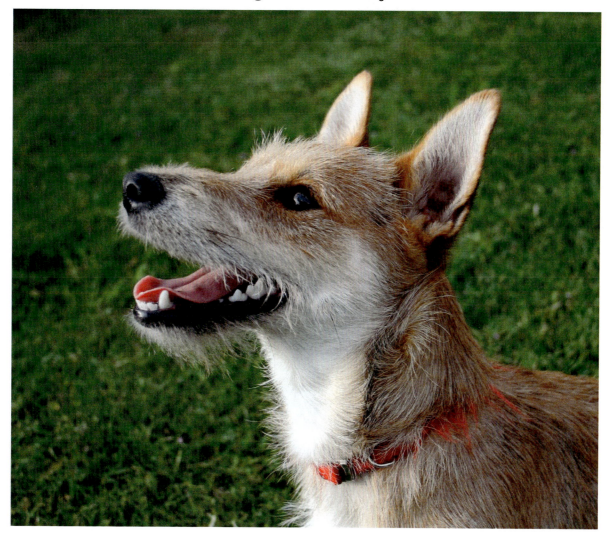

xiv

1. I went outside to walk the _____.

2. What do you do with one?

3. Who has them?

4. Why do people have them?

5. Pretend to pet one.

Naming Functional Objects

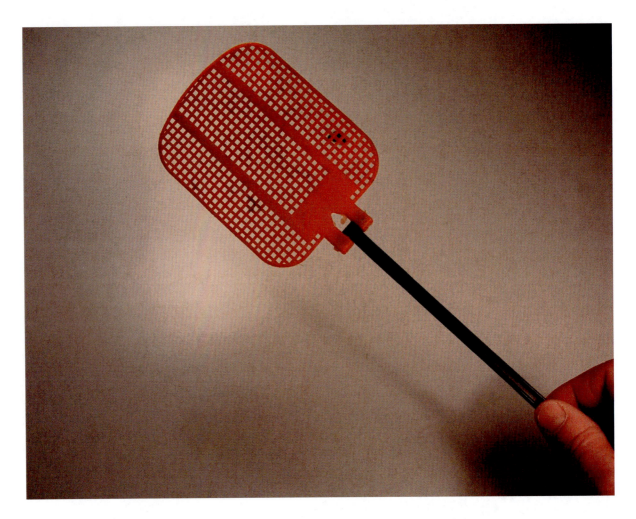

xv

1. There are too many flies on the picnic table. I better go get the fly _____.

2. When do you use it?

3. What do you do with it?

4. What time of year do you need it?

5. Pretend to use one.

Naming Functional Objects

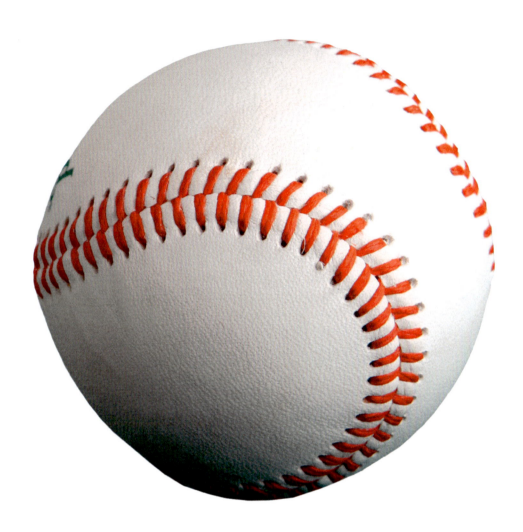

xvi

1. The little boy swung the bat and hit the _____.

2. What do you do with it?

3. Who uses it?

4. Where do you use it?

5. Pretend to throw one.

Naming Functional Objects

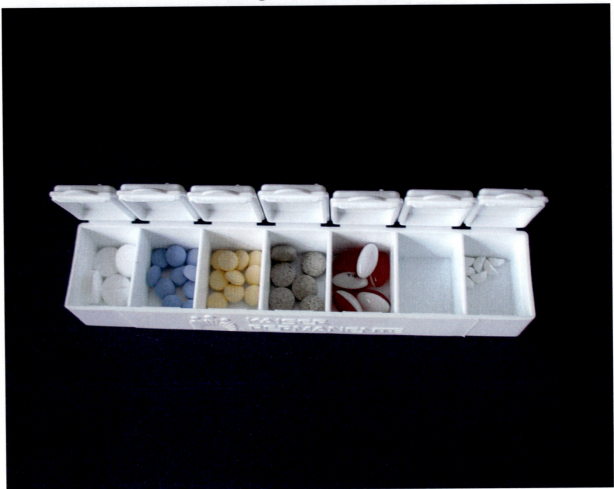

xvii

1. Time to take my _____.

2. Where do you get it?

3. Who gives it to you?

4. Who uses it?

5. Pretend to take some.

Naming Functional Objects

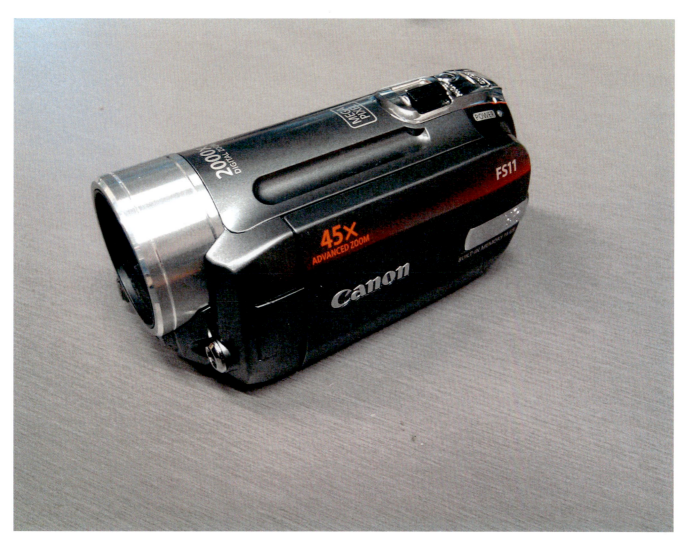

1. We are going to an award ceremony. I can't forget the _____!

2. Why do you use it?

3. What does it do?

4. When do you use it?

5. Pretend to use one.

Naming Functional Objects

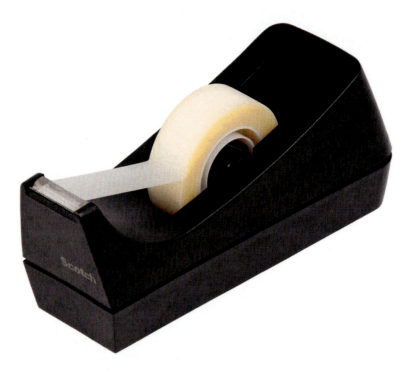

xix

1. To wrap this birthday present, I'll need a lot of scotch_____.

2. Where do you keep it?

3. What do you put it on?

4. What does it do?

5. Pretend you are using some.

Naming Functional Objects

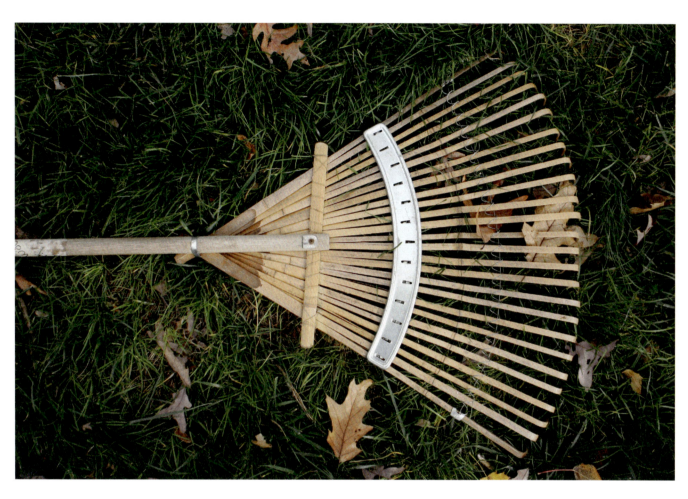

xx

1. The lawn is covered in leaves. I need to _____.

2. What is it used for?

3. Who uses it?

4. When do you use it?

5. Pretend to use one.

Naming Functional Objects

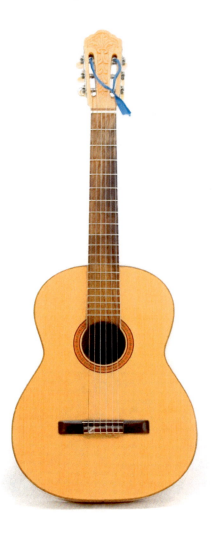

xxi

1. I'm so proud of myself because I learned how to play the _____.

2. What does it do?

3. Who plays it?

4. Where would you see one?

5. Pretend to play one.

Naming Functional Objects

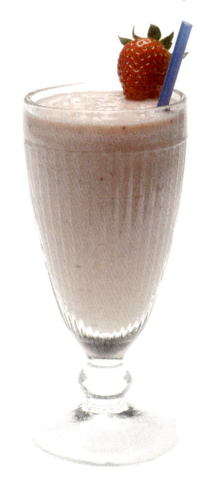

1. For dessert, I'm going to order a strawberry _____.

2. What do you do with it?

3. When do you have one?

4. Where could you get one?

5. Pretend you are drinking one.

Naming Functional Objects

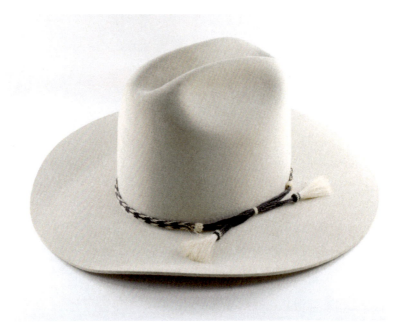

xxiii

1. The country music singer always wore a _____.

2. Where do you wear it?

3. Who wears it?

4. Why would you wear it?

5. Pretend to put one on.

Naming Functional Objects

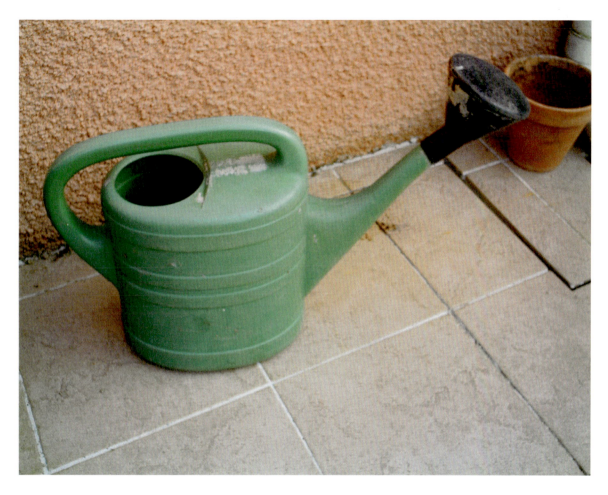

xxiv

1. It hasn't rained in awhile. I'll water the plants with my _____.

2. What time of year do you use it?

3. Who uses it?

4. Why do you use it?

5. Pretend to use one.

Naming Functional Objects

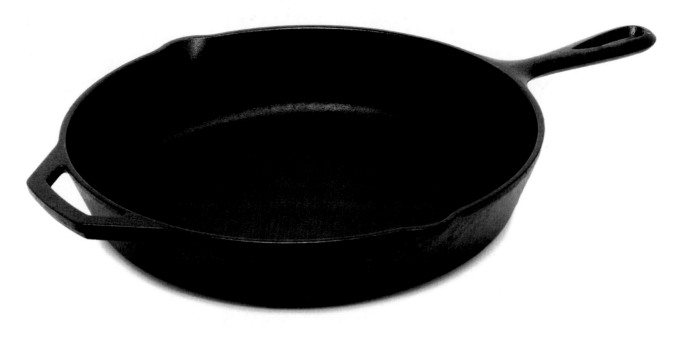

xxv

1. I'm going to cook some scrambled eggs in the frying _____.

2. Where do you use it?

3. What is it used for?

4. Who uses it?

5. Pretend you are cooking with one.

Naming Functional Objects

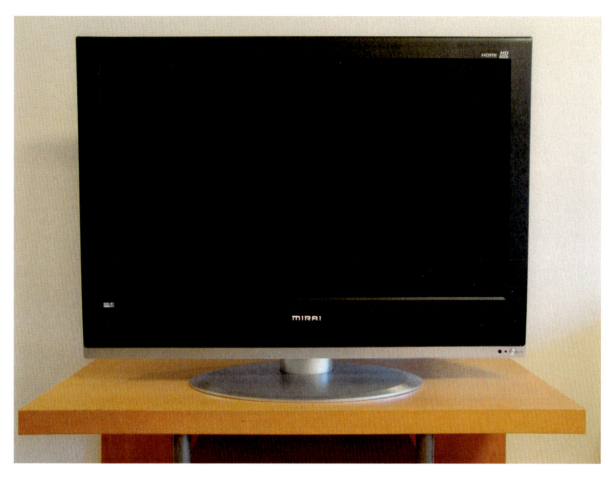

xxvi

1. I'm going to relax and watch some _____.

2. What do you do with it?

3. When do you use it?

4. Who uses it?

5. Pretend you are changing the channel on it.

Naming Functional Objects

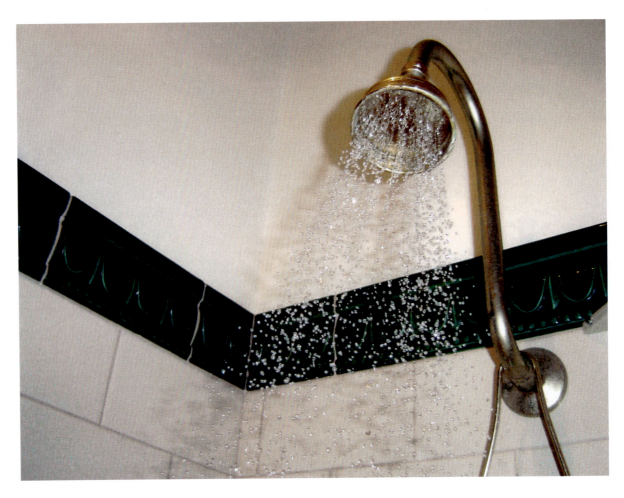

xxvii

1. In the morning, I got up and took a _____.

2. Where do you find one?

3. Why do you use it?

4. When do you use it?

5. Pretend you are using it.

Naming Functional Objects

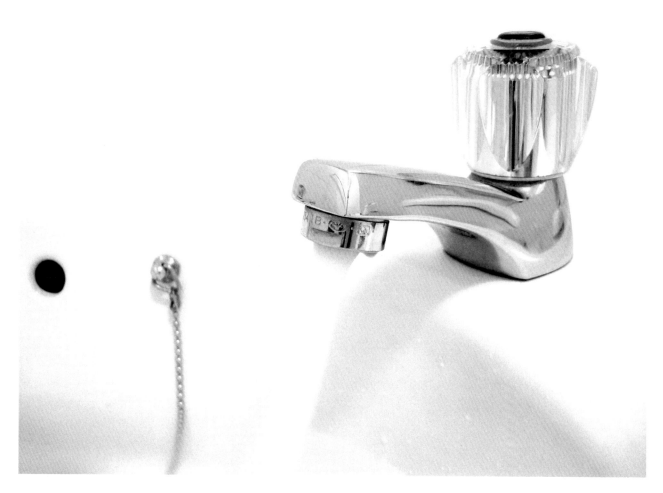

xxviii

1. Turn on the bathroom _____.

2. Where do you find it?

3. How do you use it?

4. What do you do with it?

5. Pretend you are using it.

Naming Functional Objects

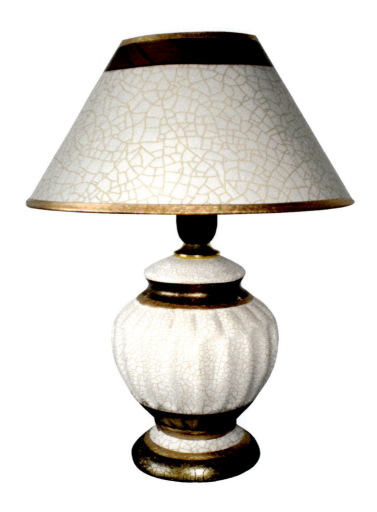

xxix

1. It is too dark in here. Please turn on the _____.

2. Where do you find one?

3. What does it do?

4. When do you use it?

5. Pretend you are turning one on.

Naming Functional Objects

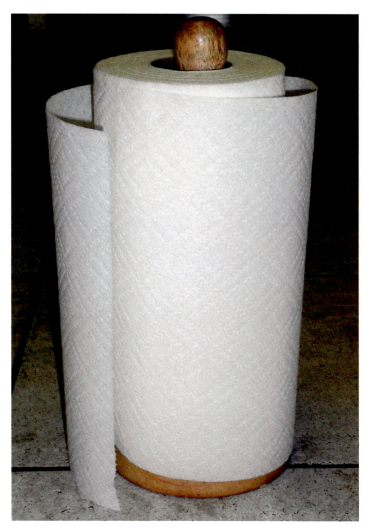

xxx

1. Whoops! I just made a big mess. I'd better get a _____.

2. Where do you keep it?

3. What do you do with it?

4. When do you use it?

5. Pretend you are using one.

Naming Functional Objects

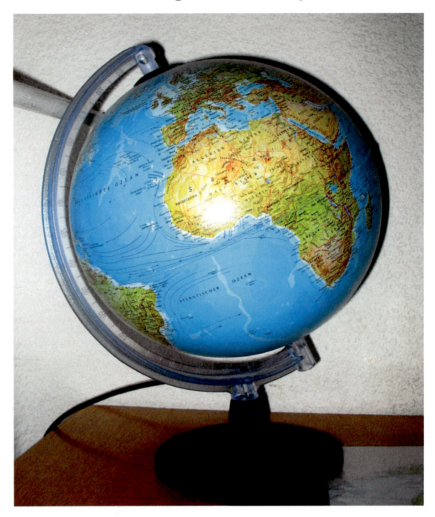

xxxi

1. I'm not sure where that country is. Let me see if I can find it on this _____.

2. Where would you find one?

3. Who uses them?

4. What are they for?

5. Pretend you are using one.

Naming Functional Objects

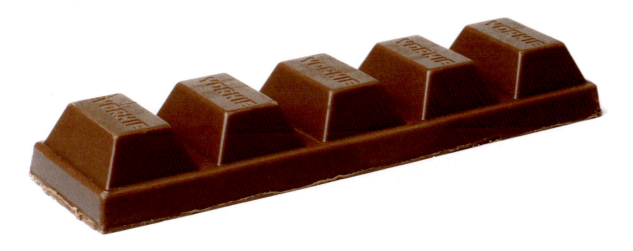

xxxii

1. Nothing makes me feel better than a piece of _____.

2. What do you do with it?

3. Who uses it?

4. When do you eat it?

5. Pretend you are eating it.

Naming Functional Objects

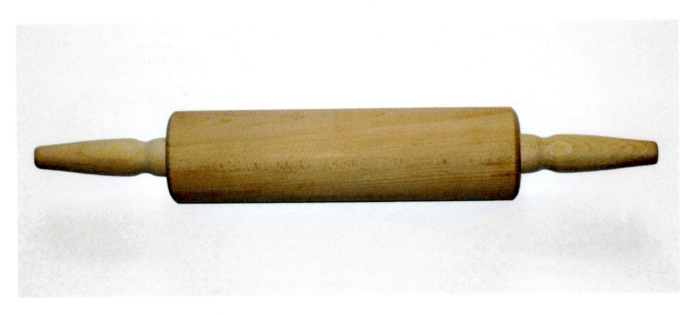

xxxiii

1. I'm going to flatten this dough by using a _____.

2. Where do you keep it?

3. What do you do with it?

4. Who uses it?

5. Pretend you are using one.

Naming Functional Objects

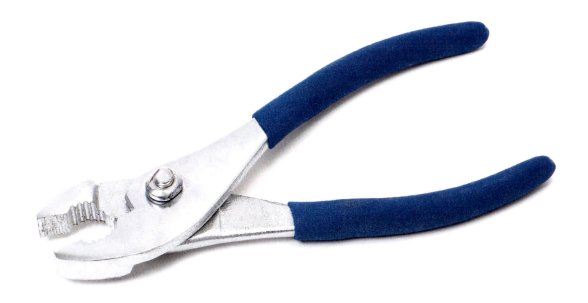

xxxiv

1. Please hand me a pair of _____.

2. What do you use it for?

3. When do you use it?

4. Who uses it?

5. Pretend you are using them.

Naming Functional Objects

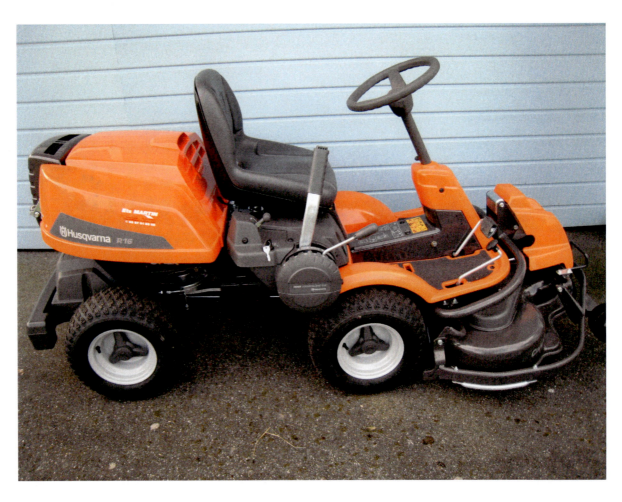

/xxxv

1. The grass is getting tall, I'd better use my ride on _____.

2. What do you use it for?

3. Where do you keep one?

4. Who uses one?

5. Pretend you are using one.

Naming Functional Objects

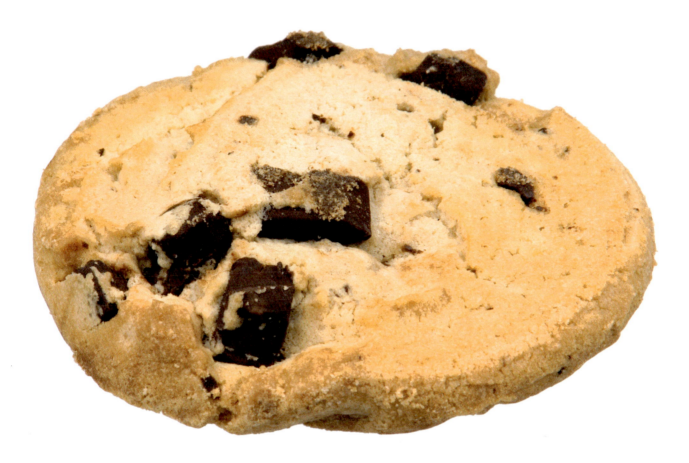

xxxvi

1. I just baked a batch of chocolate chip _____.

2. Who eats them?

3. When do you bake them?

4. Where do you keep them?

5. Pretend you are eating one.

Naming Functional Objects

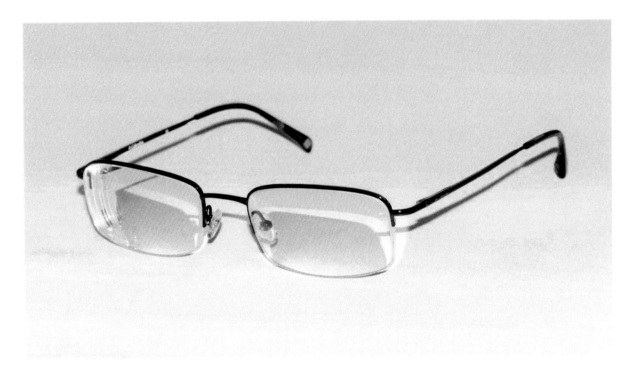

xxxvii

1. I can't read that size print without my _____.

2. Who wears them?

3. What are they for?

4. When do people wear them?

5. Pretend you are putting on a pair.

Naming Functional Objects

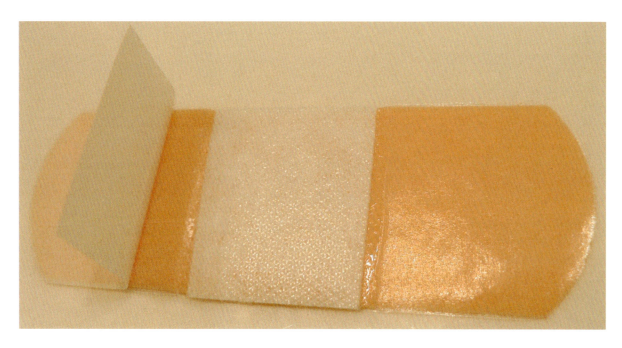

xxxviii

1. Ouch! I cut my finger. I need a _____.

2. Why do you use one?

3. Who uses them?

4. Where do you keep them?

5. Pretend you are putting one on.

Naming Functional Objects

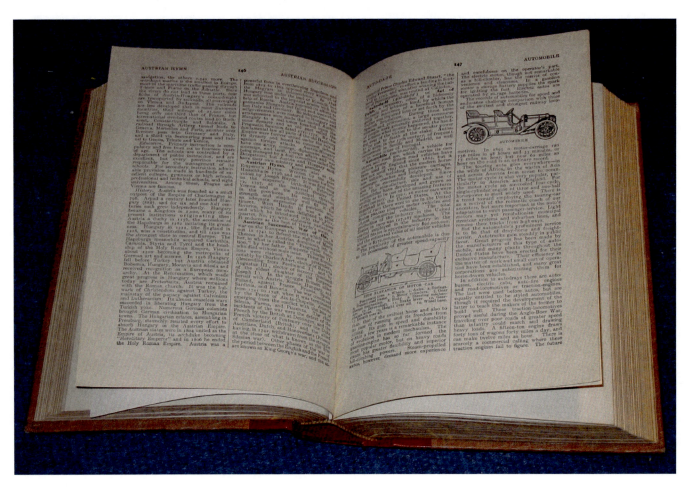

xxxix

1. I'm going to sit down and read a good _____.

2. Where would you find one?

3. What do you do with it?

4. Who uses it?

5. Pretend you are reading one.

Naming Functional Objects

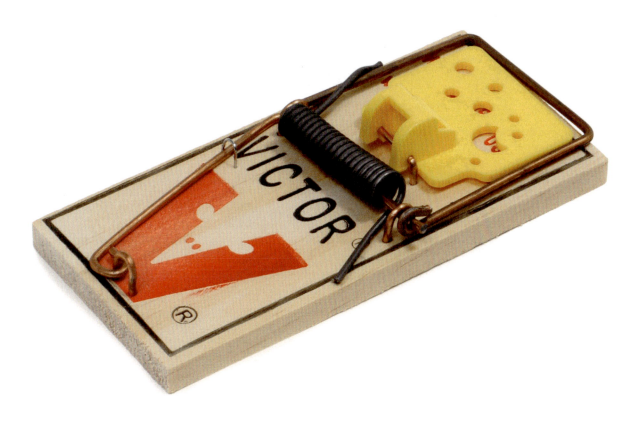

xl

1. Oh no, I hear scratching in the attic. I better set some _____.

2. Why do you use them?

3. What do they do?

4. Where would you put one?

5. Pretend you are setting one.

Naming Functional Objects

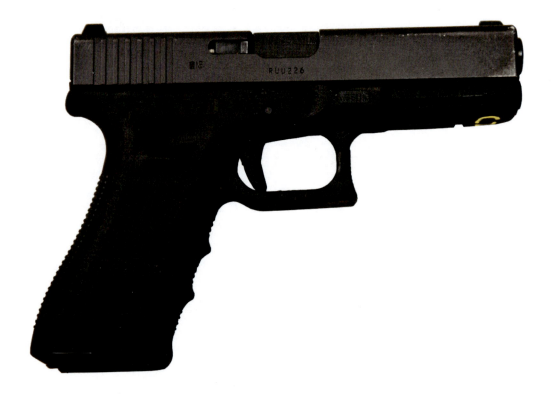

xli

1. Do you believe there should be background checks to buy a _____?

2. What is it used for?

3. Who uses it?

4. Why would you use one?

5. Pretend you are using one.

Naming Functional Objects

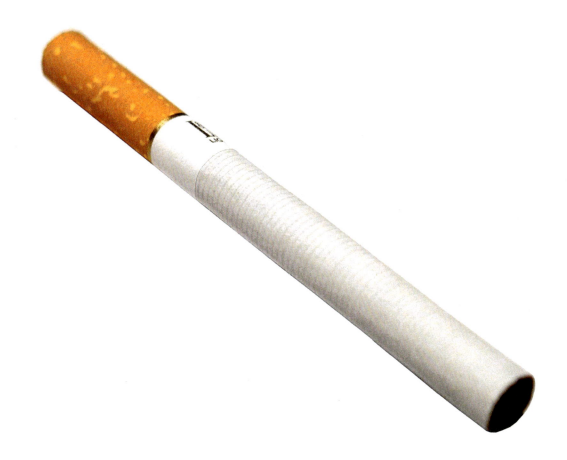

xlii

1. He asked if he could bum a _____.

2. What do you do with it?

3. Who uses it?

4. Why do people use them?

5. Pretend you are smoking one.

Naming Functional Objects

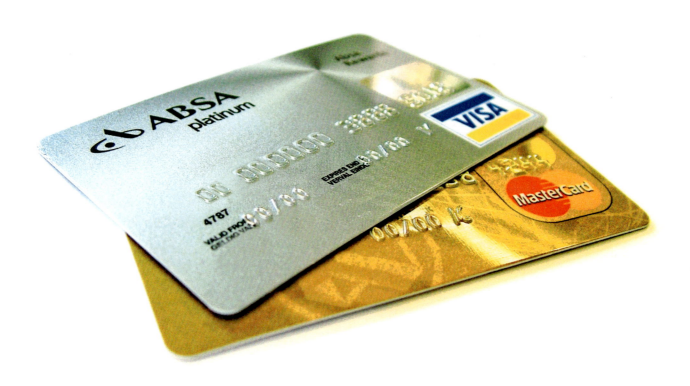

xliii

1. I'll just put that purchase on my _____.

2. Where do you keep them?

3. What do you use them for?

4. When would you use them?

5. Pretend you are handing somebody one.

Naming Functional Objects

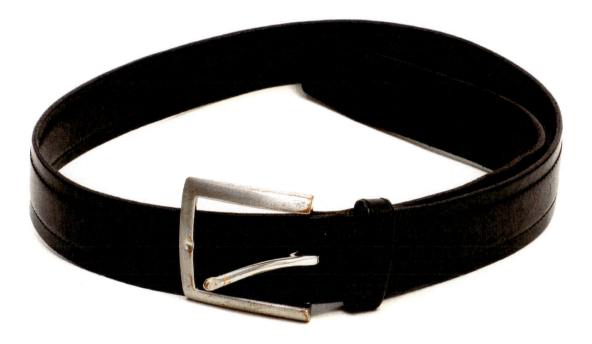

xliv

1. Time to tighten your_____.

2. Where do you wear it?

3. Why would you wear it?

4. Who wears it?

5. Pretend you are putting one on.

Naming Functional Objects

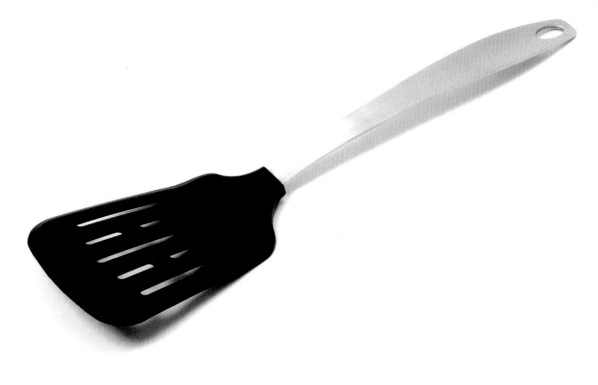

xlv

1. I need to turn over the pancakes with this _____.

2. What do you do with it?

3. When would you use it?

4. Where do you keep it?

5. Pretend you are using one.

Naming Functional Objects

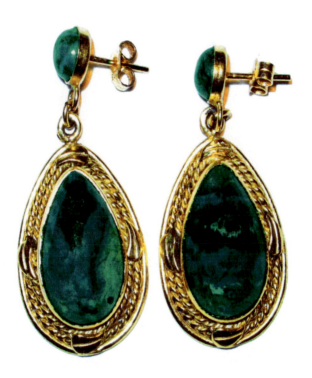

xlvi

1. I bought a new pair of _____.

2. Where do you wear them?

3. Who wears them?

4. When do you wear them?

5. Pretend you are putting them in.

Naming Functional Objects

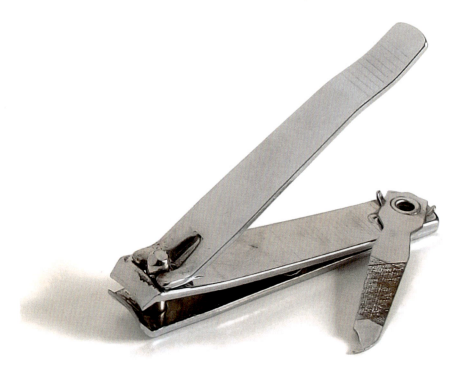

xlvii

1. I need to trim my nails. I better use the _____.

2. Where do you keep them?

3. What do you do with them?

4. Who uses them?

5. Pretend you are using them.

Naming Functional Objects

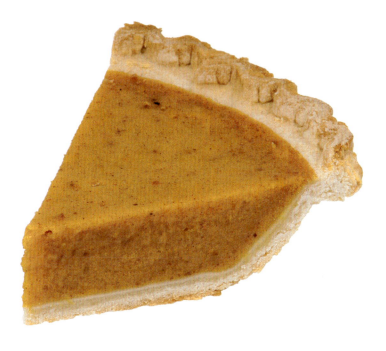

xlviii

1. I'm going to have another slice of pumpkin_____.

2. What time of year do you eat it?

3. Where could you buy it?

4. How do you make it?

5. Pretend you are taking a bite.

Naming Functional Objects

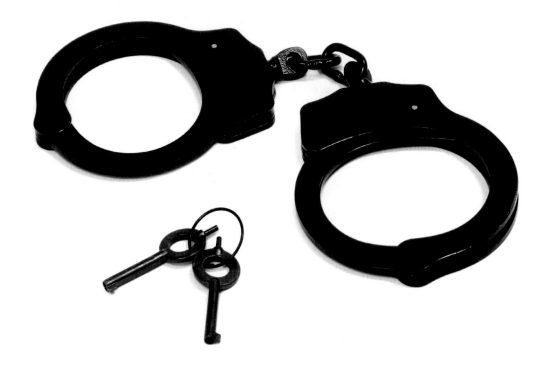

xlix

1. The prisoner had to wear a pair of _____.

2. Who uses them?

3. Where do you find them?

4. What are they for?

5. Pretend have them on.

Naming Functional Objects

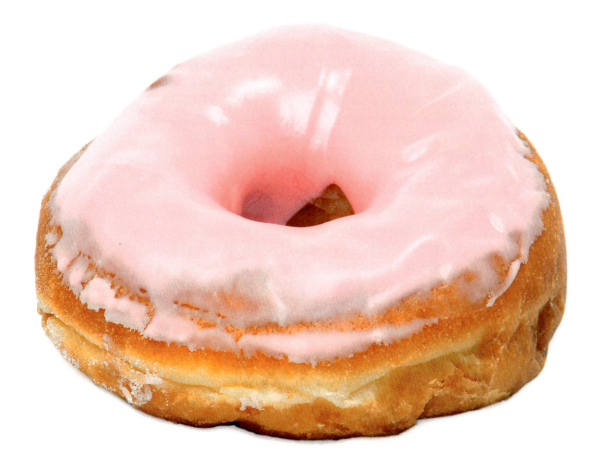

1. I would like a pink glazed _____.

2. When do you eat it?

3. What do you do with it?

4. Where do you find it?

5. Pretend you are taking a bite of one.

Rote Naming

These are more automatic categories. Ask your partner to say each item. If it is too difficult, have them read it or sing it with you first and then on their own. (Try covering up the other letters as you go or pointing to make it easier). Memory, rhythm and repetition contribute to improve expressive language abilities for these exercises.

ABCs:

A B C D E F G H I J K L M

N O P Q R S T U V W X Y Z

Counting:

1 2 3 4 5 6 7 8 9 10 11 12 13

14 15 16 17 18 19 20 21 22 23

24 25 26 27 28 29 30

Rote Naming

Days of the week:

Sunday

Monday

Tuesday

Wednesday

Thursday

Friday

Saturday

Months of the year

January	**July**
February	**August**
March	**September**
April	**October**
May	**November**
June	**December**

Convergent Naming

Descriptions:

In this exercise, read the description of the item. Try to name the item described. If the answer doesn't come after listening to or reading the description, use the phrase at the end to help retrieve the word.

1. These go in your mouth. Not everybody has them. They can be partial or full. They help you chew. You use adhesive like Fixodent with them. You take them out at night.

Before I eat this steak dinner, I better put in my _____.

2. This is something you eat. You need a spoon. It can be thick and creamy or have vegetables in it. It can be served as a meal or an appetizer. It is especially good on a cold day.

I'd like a bowl of chicken noodle _____.

3. This is a drink. The cold kind is very popular in the South. The hot kind is very popular in England and for breakfast. It can be sweet or unsweet. It needs to be brewed. I can be served hot or cold.

Would you like some lemon in your _____?

4. This is a vegetable. It is green. Some people like it and some people strongly dislike it. George Bush hated it. You can eat it raw or cooked. You can serve it in a casserole.

The soup is green. It must be cream of _____.

Convergent Naming

1. This is usually on shirts or pants and helps clasp clothing together. If you lose one you will need to sew on another one. They are small and round and have either two or four small holes.

That little baby is cute as a _____.

2. This is a fruit. It can be red or green. They grow on a vine and in bunches. Wine is made from them.

The fruit basket had apples, oranges and a bunch of green _____.

3. This is something you read. People often order a subscription to get one every week or month. You can buy them at the grocery store or a news-stand. Their sales have gone down because of the internet and mobile devices but you can also read them on a computer.

I'm thinking of buying a subscription to Time _____.

4. This is a type of shoe. You wear it mostly in the summer especially at the beach. They are open except for a strap which can be cloth, plastic or leather.

On the beach, I wore a pair of flip _____.

Convergent Naming

1. This is a vegetable. It can be yellow, red or white. You can eat it raw or on a salad or hamburger. You can also cook it and add it to all kinds of dishes. When you cut it, it can make you cry.

   The recipe calls for a Vidalia _____.

2. This is a place. Many people are scared to go here. There are chairs that recline and small sinks to spit in. It is an office of a medical professional. Sometimes you go just for a cleaning and other times you may need a filling.

   Every six months, you should go to the _____.

3. This is an item of clothing. Not many people wear one. You would see it on Halloween. Magicians, super heroes and vampires might wear one. It attaches around your neck or shoulders and hangs down your back.

   Superman wears a red _____.

4. This object usually has a rubber end with a small handle. You would find one at the library, passport desk at customs and the post office. You press the rubber end on a sponge filled with ink and then press it onto paper to produce an image.

   The Italian custom's agent marked my passport with a _____.

Convergent Naming

1. This is something you would find at a party. It has a string so you can hang it up high. When you play with it, you wear a blindfold and swing a stick. They are filled with candy. The goal is to hit it until it breaks.

    The kids cheered when candy poured out of the donkey _____.

2. This is a religious holiday in the spring. On this day, women and girls wear fancy dresses and some cities have parades. Children believe that a bunny hides eggs filled with candy. Children also decorate eggs for the bunny to hide. People often get together with family and serve a ham.

    Christians believe that Jesus was resurrected on _____.

3. This is an organ that pumps blood. It is also a shape that symbolises love. You would see lots of these on Valentine's day decorations and cards.

    When my boyfriend dumped me, he broke my _____.

4. This is a type of bird. They are found in the rainforest. They are very colorful. People can keep them as pets. You might see one on a pirate's shoulder. They can be taught to talk.

    Stop repeating everything I say like a _____.

Divergent Naming

Broad Categories with Subcategories:

The goal of these exercises is to name items that belong in each category. These are broad categories that are broken down into subcategories to increase naming ability. Encourage visualisation of places, gestures and use phonemic cues (the first sound of the desired word) to increase ability to name items in each category.

U.S. States

A-Z: Use the alphabet to help think of different States. Go through the alphabet and try to name a state for each letter that applies.

Visualize driving East to West across the U.S. and name states as you go

Visualize driving North to South on both coasts and name the states along the way

1st 13 Colonies

States that begin with the letter M

Southern States

States you have lived in

States you've visited

Animals

pets

jungle animals

forest animals

A-Z (try to name an animal for each letter of the alphabet)

farm animals

zoo animals

animals smaller than a basket ball

animals larger than a person

extinct animals

Divergent Naming

Broad Categories with subcategories

Clothing
footwear

bottoms

undergarments

tops

neckwear

hands

head

woman's

men

fancy dress

casual

inappropriate

beach

winter

generational style: 20s, 30s, 40s, 50s, 60s, 70s, 80s, 90s.....

Furniture
dining Room

living Room

bedroom

patio

storage

types of chairs

office

Divergent Naming

Broad Categories with subcategories

Sports

professional

woman's

outdoor

indoor

water

snow

team sports

individual sports

adrenaline sports (sky diving etc.)

combat

Olympic

sports people bet on

sports you have played

sports you like to watch

Movies

westerns

horror

action

comedy

drama

romance

Oscar winners

your favorites

kids

least favorites

Divergent Naming

Categories:

Say as many items as you can that belong in each category. Start with three in each category and work up to as many as you can think of.

Things you recycle	Things you buy at a Bakery
Things you bring camping	Types of soup
School subjects	Religions
Last names	Charities
School subjects	Ethnic food
Musical instruments	Condiments
Alcoholic drinks	Cleaning supplies
Famous works of art	Vacation destinations
Flowers	Baby supplies
Snack foods	Insects
Actors	Ice cream flavors
Dinosaurs	Reasons for a party
Headache medicines	Pool toys
Wars	City transportation

Divergent Naming

Medical professions	Blue collar jobs
Vitamins/Supplements	Ways to cover up baldness
Facial hair	Bands
Detergents	European Cities
U.S. Cities	Famous beaches
Cereal brands	Things served at a BBQ
Italian foods	Southern food
California Cities	Fast food restaurants
Luxury cars	American cars
Antique car makes	Acts in a circus
Painting supplies	Hair styles
Places to go on a date	Natural disasters
Parts of a car	Types of bills
Banks	Shoes
Hats	Make up
Music genres	Things you bring to the beach

Divergent Naming

Fattening Foods	Diet foods
Seafood	Things you put on a salad
Dances	Late night talk show hosts
Morning shows	News anchors
Playground equipment	Stuffed animals
Pest you call an exterminator for	Berries
Authors	Electronics
Dog breeds	Trees
Building materials	Small appliances
Large appliances	Outdoor toys
Arts and crafts materials	Shipping companies
Brands of soap	Table settings
Breakfast foods	Cookies
Muffins	Flowers
Yard tools	European Countries
Asian Countries	Countries in the Middle East

Divergent Naming

Countries in South America

Precious stones

Foods made from potatoes

Breakfast restaurants

Mexican food dishes

Mobile phone service providers

Cheeses

Microwavable foods

Brands of chocolate

Department stores

Rides at an amusement park

Meats

Birds

Juices

Weapons

Jewelry

Precious metals

Cold remedies

Vegetables

Clothing materials

Cable companies

Oceans

Candy

Spices

Foods sold at a fair

Hardware stores

Road signs

Reptiles

Dairy products

Illegal drugs

Melodic Intonation Exercises

The Right Hemisphere of the brain controls music and rhythm and can be a powerful tool to help the left hemisphere recover from a stroke and increase expressive language. These exercises focus on singing and rhythm to increase fluency. Pick songs or rhymes that are familiar and flow naturally. Have your partner sing them as much as they can from memory instead of reading them. It should be a memory and singing exercise opposed to a reading exercise. Sing with your partner to help cue and initiate the song. Most likely, some of the lyrics to the songs will need to be relearned as they aren't know by heart by everyone.

Twinke Twinkle Little Star

by Jane Taylor

Twinkle Twinkle Little Star

How I wonder what you are

Up above the world so high

Like a diamond in the sky

Twinkle Twinkle Little Star

How I wonder what you are

Rock-a-bye Baby

Rock-a-bye baby, on the tree top

When the wind blows, the cradle will rock,

When the bough breaks, the cradle will fall,

And down will come baby, cradle and all.

Melodic Intonation Exercises

Mary Had a Little Lamb

Sarah Josepha Hale

Mary had a little lamb,
Little lamb, little lamb,
Mary had a little lamb,
Its fleece was white as snow

And everywhere that Mary went,
Mary went, Mary went,
Everywhere that Mary went
The lamb was sure to go

It followed her to school one day
School one day, school one day
It followed her to school one day
Which was against the rules.

It made the children laugh and play,
Laugh and play, laugh and play,
It made the children laugh and play
To see a lamb at school

Melodic Intonation Exercises

Star Spangled Banner

Francis Scott Key

O say can you see, by the dawn's early light,

What so proudly we hailed at the twilight's last gleaming,

Whose broad stripes and bright stars through the perilous fight,

O'er the ramparts we watched, were so gallantly streaming?

And the rocket's red glare, the bombs bursting in air,

Gave proof through the night that our flag was still there;

O say does that star-spangled banner yet wave,

O'er the land of the free and the home of the brave?

Yankee Doodle

Yankee Doodle went to town

A-riding on a pony,

Stuck a feather in his cap

And called it macaroni'.

Yankee Doodle keep it up,

Yankee Doodle dandy,

Mind the music and the step,

And with the girls be handy.

Melodic Intonation Exercises

You're a Grand Old Flag
George M. Cohan

You're a grand old flag
You're a high flying flag
And forever in peace may you wave.
You're the emblem of
The land I love.
The home of the free and the brave.
Every heart beats true for the red white and blue
Where there's never a boast or a brag.
Should old acquaintance be forgot.
Keep your eye on the grand old flag.

America The Beautiful
Words by Katharine Lee Bates
Melody by Samuel Ward

O beautiful for spacious skies,
For amber waves of grain,
For purple mountain majesty,
Above the fruited plain!
America! America!
God shed his grace on thee,
And crowned thy good with brotherhood,
From sea to shining sea!

Melodic Intonation Exercises

Jingle Bells

James Lord Pierpont

Dashing through the snow

On a one horse open sleigh

O'er the fields we go

Laughing all the way

Bells on Bob tails ring

Making spirits bright

What fun it is to laugh and sing

A sleighing song tonight

Oh jingle bells, jingle bells

Jingle all the way

Oh, what fun it is to ride

On a one horse open sleigh

Oh jingle bells, jingle bells

Jingle all the way

Oh, what fun it is to ride

On a one horse open sleigh

Melodic Intonation Exercises

Deck the Halls

Thomas Oliphant

Deck the hall with boughs of holly,

Fa la la la la la la la la

Tis the season to be jolly,

Fa la la la la la la la la

Don we now our gay apparel,

Troll the ancient Christmas carol,

Fa la la la la la la la la

See the blazing yule before us,

Fa la la la la la la la la

Strike the harp and join the chorus.

Fa la la la la la la la la

Follow me in merry measure

While I tell of Christmas treasure,

Fa la la la la la la la la

Fast away the old year passes,

Fa la la la la la la la la

Hail the new, ye lads and lasses!

Fa la la la la la la la la

Sing we joyous all together,

Heedless of the wind and weather,

Fa la la la la la la la la

Functional Writing

Make Copies of these forms and practice writing personal information.

Personal Information

First Name:	
Middle Name:	
Last Name:	

Date of Birth	
Social Security Number:	
Address:	

Phone number:		
Cell number:		
Emergency Contact Name:		
Emergency Contact phone #		

Additional Information:

Work history:	
Insurance Carrier	
Policy Number:	
Group Number:	

Medical Information

First Name:		Last Name:	

Date of Birth	
Social Security Number:	
Address:	

Phone number:		
Cell number:		
Emergency Contact Name:		
Emergency Contact phone #		

Additional Information:

Medications	
Insurance Carrier	
Policy Number:	
Group Number:	
Medical History:	

Family Information

First Name: **Last Name:**

Date of Birth	
Social Security Number:	
Address:	

Phone number:		
Cell number:		
Emergency Contact:		
Emergency Contact phone #		

Family Information:

Spouse		Phone number:	
Children:		Phone number:	
		Phone number:	
		Phone number:	
Siblings		Phone number:	
		Phone number:	
		Phone number:	
		Phone number:	
		Phone number:	
		Phone number:	
Father's name			
Mother's name			

Job Application

Date_____

Name _____ Social Security # _____
     First   Middle   Last

Address

_____

_____

_____

Current Phone: home:_____**Cell:**_____

E-Mail Address: _____

Position Desired:_____

What are your dates of availability?_____

Date of Birth:____/____/____   Please Circle: Male / Female

Do you possess a valid driver's license? Yes[ ] No[ ] Which state? _____

Drivers license#_____

Are you legally authorized to be employed in the USA? Yes[ ] No[ ]

Have you ever been convicted of a criminal offense? Yes[ ] No[ ] If yes, please explain
_____

Education Information
Circle your present year in school: High School 3 4 College 1 2 3 4 Graduate 1 2 3

	School Name, City, and State	Course of Study/Major	Graduated	Degree Received
High School			Yes [ ] No [ ]	
College			Yes [ ] No [ ]	
Other			Yes [ ] No [ ]	

Employment History
List all work experience beginning with your **current or most recent position**.

Company Name _____ Employed from_____ to _____
Address
_____

_____
Name & Title of Immediate Supervisor_____
Telephone_____
Your Title _____
Reason for leaving_____
Description of
Responsibilities_____

_____

Company Name _____ Employed from_____ to _____
Address
_____

_____
Name & Title of Immediate Supervisor_____
Telephone_____
Your Title _____
Reason for leaving_____
Description of
Responsibilities_____

_____

Company Name _____ Employed from_____ to _____
Address
_____

_____
Name & Title of Immediate Supervisor_____
Telephone_____
Your Title _____
Reason for leaving_____
Description of
Responsibilities_____

_____

Function of Items

Explain what each item is used for.

elevator	soda machine	chainsaw
shoe horn	remote control	megaphone
telescope	slot machine	ATM
broom	chair	clock
door bell	keys	microwave
pen	pillow	refrigerator
pacifier	harmonica	microphone
scissors	whistle	bus
dump truck	wig	iron
umbrella	metal detector	hanger
zipper	faucet	gasoline
fishing net	light switch	curtains
hair scrunchy	head phones	subway
salad spinner	cork screw	sandpaper
wrench	hammer	treadmill
tennis racket	Neosporin	mouthwash
kitty litter	leash	helmet
baby aspirin	girdle	tweezers

Function of Items

Explain what each item is used for.

cannon	ashtray	spoon
straw	aluminum foil	tongs
propane tank	tongs	ladder
dog tags	Christmas lights	dental floss
tissues	baby stroller	Easter basket
Windex	cigar	water fountain
doggy bag	cane	call bell
stamp	computer mouse	camera
escalator	cash register	credit card
dryer sheet	sponge	baby powder
grocery cart	paper towel	shaving cream
car jack	fuse box	rain gutters
shingles	stair rail	Coinstar
shower poof	nail file	mover's dolly
thermometer	mouth guard	bike helmet
laxative	scarf	chap stick
visor	jumper cables	perfume

What Questions

1. What drink comes from cows? _____

2. What burns on a wick and melts wax? _____

3. What show has multiple acts including acrobats, elephants and clowns?

   _____

4. What do you eat at the movies? _____

5. What insect bites you and makes you itchy? _____

6. What is a permanent ink design on skin? _____

7. What material do people like on their kitchen counter tops? _____

8. What do you put on your skin to keep it moist? _____

9. What do people do in the woods with a tent? _____

10. What do you throw at a bull's eye? _____

11. What facial hair grows under the nose? _____

12. What do you wear to cover your eyes when the sun is bright? _____

13. What precious metal is the most valuable? _____

14. What do you blow up for guests to sleep on? _____

15. What do you put on the top of a wrapped present? _____

When Questions

1. When do leaves change color? _____
2. When do babies start to walk? _____
3. When should you stop at a stop light? _____
4. When do birds fly south? _____
5. When should you get an oil change? _____
6. When do people eat breakfast? _____
7. When do people retire? _____
8. When do boys have a bar mitzvah? _____
9. When is confirmation in the Catholic Church? _____
10. When do we watch fireworks? _____
11. When should you stop wearing white? _____
12. When do families get together and eat turkey? _____
13. When do you drink green beer? _____
14. When do you go to the dentist? _____
15. When do you take a shower? _____

When Questions

1. When should somebody go on a diet? _____
2. When do you go to college? _____
3. When do you drink coffee? _____
4. When do you brush your teeth? _____
5. When does the mail come? _____
6. When do you take out your dentures? _____
7. When do you go to the beach? _____
8. When do people drink champagne? _____
9. When do you vote? _____
10. When should you wear suntan lotion? _____
11. When do you go to bed? _____
12. When do you pay your mortgage? _____
13. When do you qualify for Medicare? _____
14. When did man first walk on the moon? _____
15. When do you get your driver's license? _____

Who Questions

1. Who prevents people from drowning? _____
2. Who rides in horse races? _____
3. Who drives an ambulance? _____
4. Who catches tuna and salmon? _____
5. Who creates fashion clothing? _____
6. Who creates art with marble and clay? _____
7. Who defends people accused of a crime? _____
8. Who delivers the mail? _____
9. Who treats sick animals? _____
10. Who cuts the grass and plants flowers and shrubs? _____
11. Who gives out speeding tickets? _____
12. Who kicks rowdy people out of a bar? _____
13. Who serves food at a restaurant? _____
14. Who prepares tax returns? _____
15. Who is the head administrator of a school? _____

Who Questions

1. Who takes pictures? _____
2. Who stars in movies? _____
3. Who flies an airplane? _____
4. Who helps people suffering from depression? _____
5. Who fixes water leaks? _____
6. Who travels in outer space? _____
7. Who repairs cars? _____
8. Who cleans hotel rooms? _____
9. Who adjusts your spine? _____
10. Who writes books? _____
11. Who makes meals at a restaurant? _____
12. Who performs stand up to make people laugh? _____
13. Who plays musical instruments? _____
14. Who helps you find activities when you stay at a hotel? ___
15. Who prepares medications? _____

How Questions

Explain the sequence of steps involved in completing each task.

1. How do you get a good night sleep?
2. How do you prepare to move?
3. How can you lose weight?
4. How do you iron a shirt?
5. How do you make a bed?
6. How do you plant a vegetable garden?
7. How do you baby proof a house?
8. How do you shave?
9. How do you put in contact lenses?
10. How do you take care of a lawn?
11. How do you change a tire?
12. How do you do a load of wash?
13. How do you clean a toilet?
14. Ho do you shift gears manually?
15. How do you wrap a present?

How Questions

Explain the sequence of steps involved in completing each task.

1. How do you put on a tie?
2. How do you mail a letter?
3. How do you catch a mouse?
4. How do you wash a car?
5. How do you polish silver?
6. How do you change a diaper?
7. How do you make scrambled eggs?
8. How do you take a dog for a walk?
9. How do you wash your hands?
10. How do you tie your shoe?
11. How do you make a peanut butter and jelly sandwich?
12. How do you make hotel reservations?
13. How do you pack a suitcase?
14. How do you do a somersault?
15. How do you boil an egg?

Where Questions

1. Where is the Sistine Chapel? _____

2. Where is the U.S. Capitol? _____

3. Where is San Francisco? _____

4. Where is Atlanta? _____

5. Where is the Great Barrier Reef? _____

6. Where is the Colosseum? _____

7. Where is the Eiffel Tower? _____

8. Where is Big Ben? _____

9. Where is the Empire State building? _____

10. Where is Versailles? _____

11. Where are the Great Pyramids? _____

12. Where is Berlin? _____

13. Where is the Louvre? _____

14. Where is the Grand Canyon? _____

15. Where is Maui? _____

Where Questions

1. Where do you go to borrow books? _____
2. Where did you go to high school? _____
3. Where were you born? _____
4. Where do you live? _____
5. Where do you go to renew your driver's license? _____
6. Where do you watch a sports event? _____
7. Where do you take kids play on the swings? _____
8. Where do you sail a boat? _____
9. Where does your family live? _____
10. Where do you get your hair done? _____
11. Where do you bank? _____
12. Where do you buy used items? _____
13. Where do you pray? _____
14. Where do you get a pizza? _____
15. Where do you go grocery shopping? _____

Why Questions

1. Why do you cover a swimming pool in Autumn?

2. Why do people stop at stop signs?

3. Why do people pawn an item?

4. Who do pets have id tags?

5. Why do people play the lottery?

6. Why do you buy life insurance?

7. Why do you turn the lights off when you leave a room?

8. Why do people use coupons?

9. Why do people lock their doors?

10. Why do you go to the mall?

11. Why do dogs bark?

12. Why do people carry mace?

13. Why do people have smoke alarms?

14. Why do you take multivitamins?

15. Why do you read to children?

Why Questions

1. Why do people keep life jackets on their boats?
2. Why do people buy bait?
3. Why shouldn't you drink and drive?
4. Why do people wear bug spray?
5. Why shouldn't you swim during a thunder storm?
6. Why do babies ride in car seats?
7. Why do you grease a cookie sheet?
8. Why shouldn't you use too much salt?
9. Why do people celebrate birthdays?
10. Why do you need a passport?
11. Why do people wear steel toe boots?
12. Why do people use GPS systems in their cars?
13. Why shouldn't you text and drive?
14. Why should you wear a bike helmet?
15. Why would you call a nurse for help?

Reading Aloud Exercises

Functional Sentences:
Have your partner read each sentence aloud using their finger to point to each word as they say it. Cover up the other sentences with an index card if they are distracting.

1. What time is dinner?

2. I like to go to the movies.

3. My favorite music is jazz.

4. I'm going to plant some tomatoes in the garden.

5. What would you like to watch on TV?

6. Where are my shoes?

7. When are we leaving?

8. Can you help me?

9. Who called you?

10. I'm ready to get up.

11. I'd like to see my children.

12. I'm getting hungry.

13. I need to shower.

14. I need a sweater.

15. Please turn the heat up.

Reading Aloud Exercises

1. I finished my book and need to get another one.

2. I'm going to brush and floss my teeth.

3. I'd like to make an appointment to get my hair done.

4. Let's go shopping. I need to get new shoes.

5. We are out of milk and eggs.

6. I would like pancakes for breakfast.

7. Help me get up.

8. Did the mail come yet?

9. Please call my sister and tell her I'm doing well.

10. What time is physical therapy?

11. Please get me the nurse.

12. My sheets need to be changed.

13. What is the weather going to be like tomorrow?

14. When are you coming back?

15. Please bring me some snacks.

Reading Aloud Exercises

1. After I get up in the morning, I go to breakfast and then I watch the Price is Right.

2. I would like coffee and a biscuit. I don't want any eggs today.

3. I want to read the newspaper today. There is some pretty interesting national news.

4. I know some people enjoy it but playing Bingo isn't for me.

5. My favorite season is Fall. I just love the changing leaves and apple pie.

6. Usually on Christmas, my family comes to my house. I love the commotion and watching the little ones open presents on Christmas morning.

7. I am not a cat person. I would much rather have a dog. Plus, I am allergic to cats so I can't even be around them.

Describing Picture Scenes

Have your partner tell you as much as possible about the pictures. Try not looking at the photograph before you show it to your partner to see how completely they can describe each picture. The less you know about the picture the more details they will need to tell you.

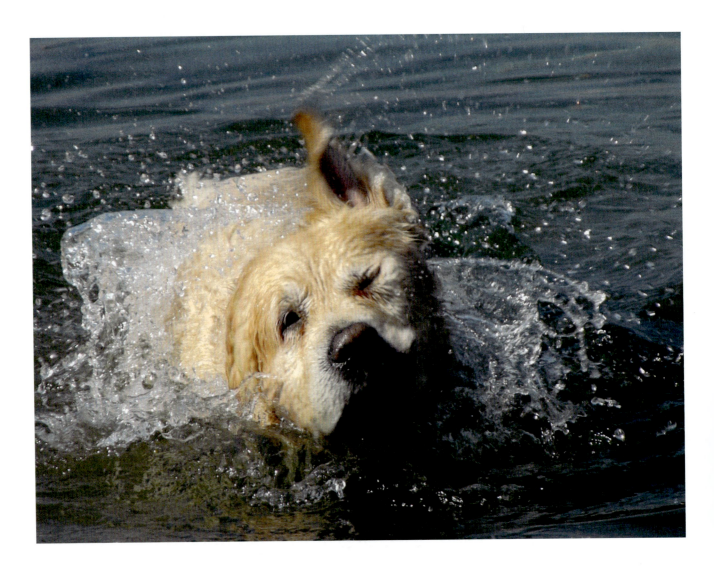

li

Describing Picture Scenes

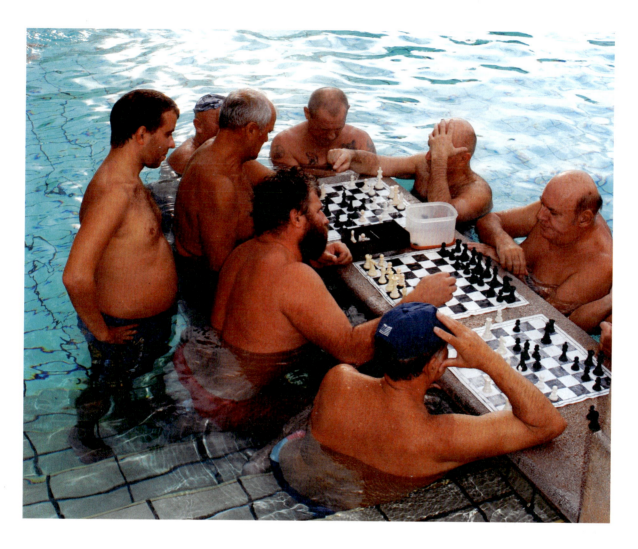

Describing Picture Scenes

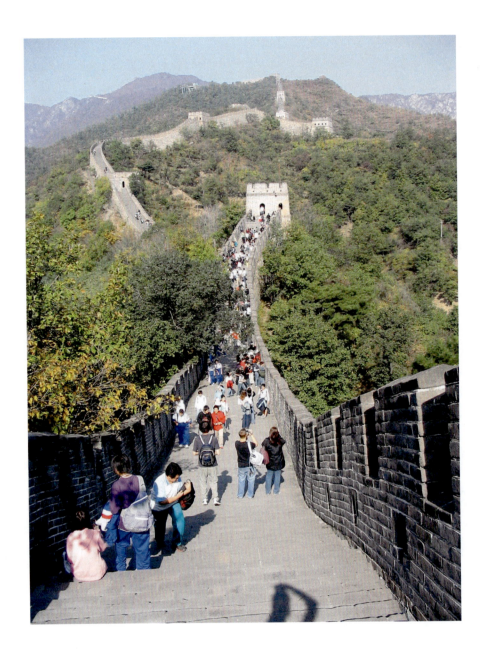

liii

Describing Picture Scenes

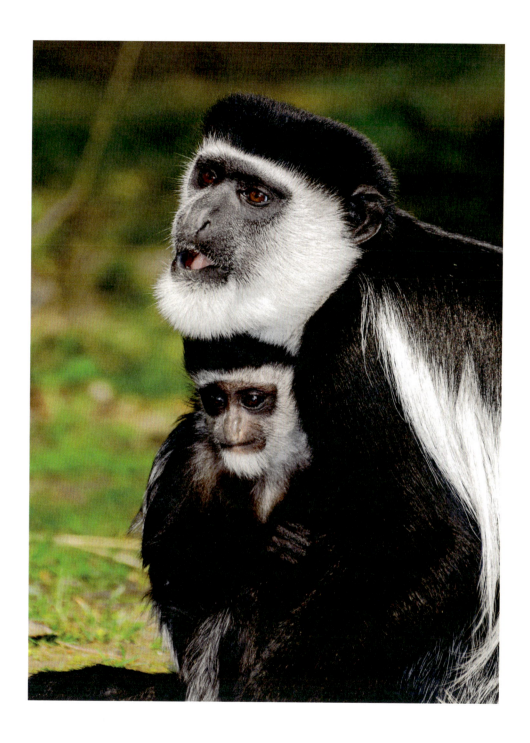

Describing Picture Scenes

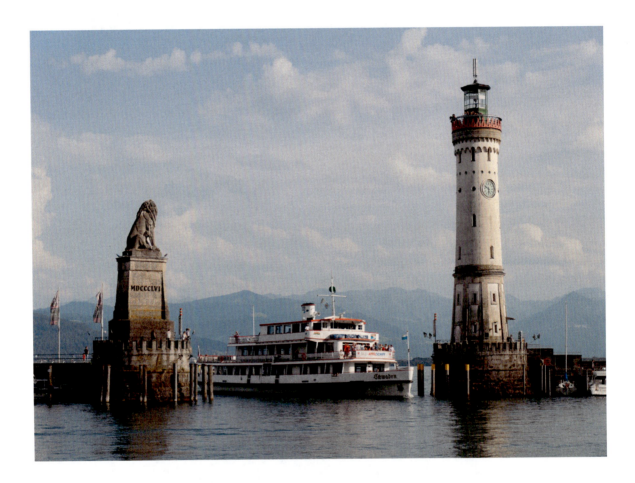

lv

Describing Picture Scenes

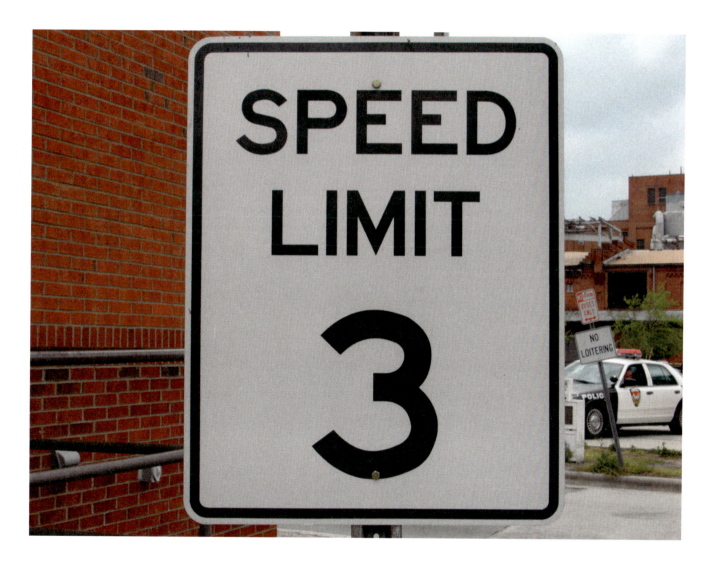

lvi

Describing Picture Scenes

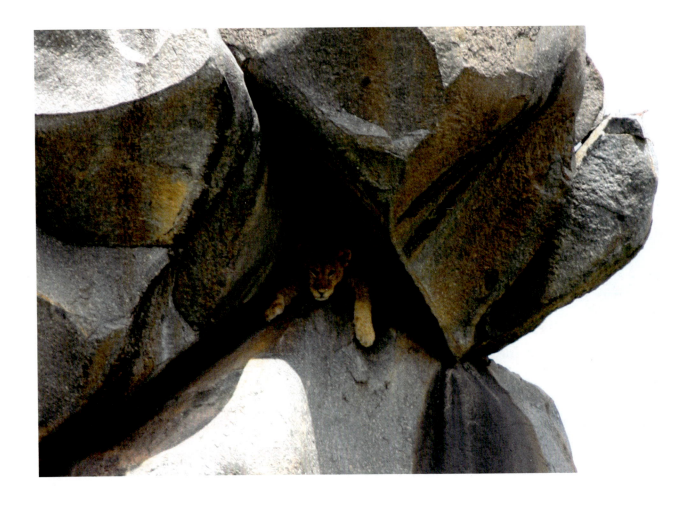

lvii

Describing Picture Scenes

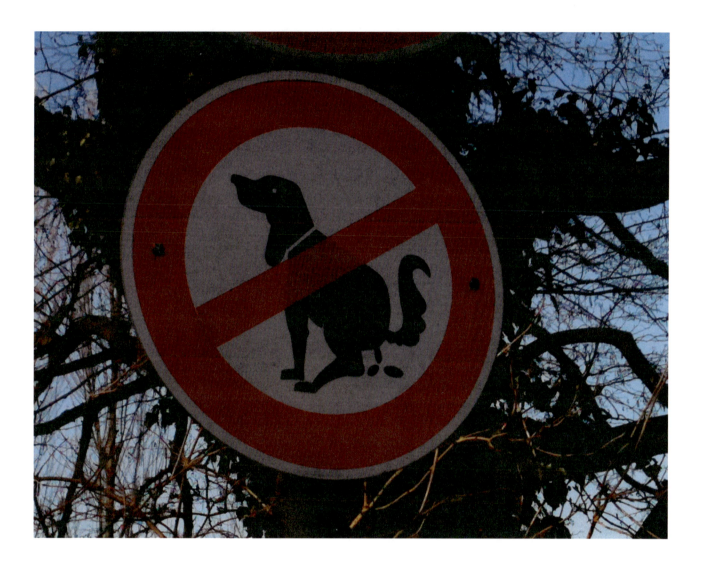

Describing Picture Scenes

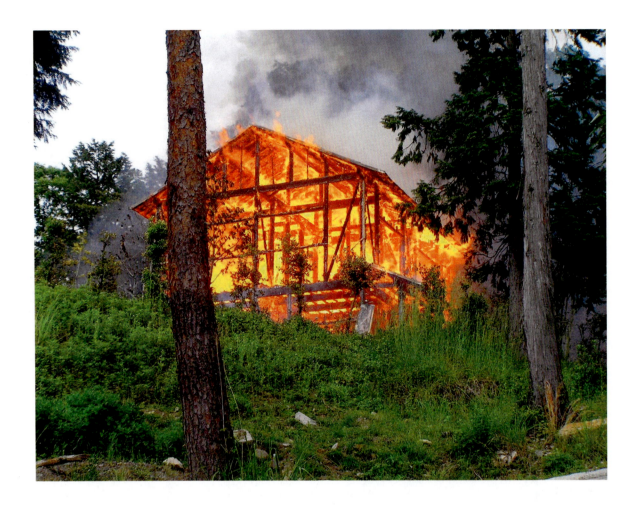

lix

Describing Picture Scenes

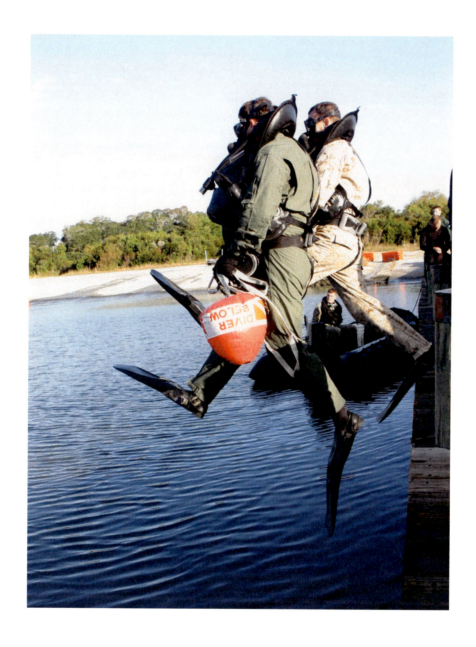

Describing Picture Scenes

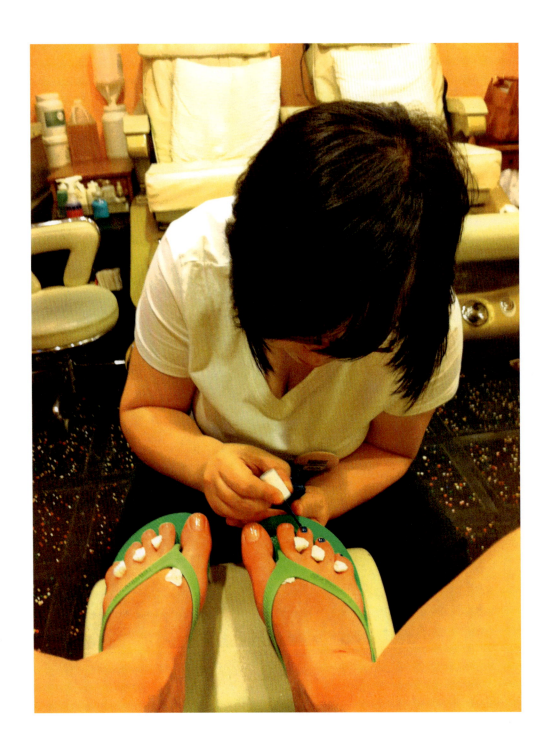

Describing Picture Scenes

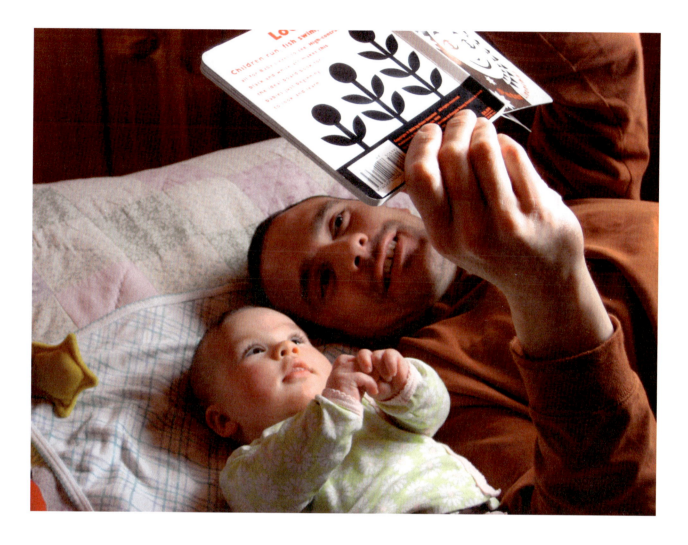

Describing Picture Scenes

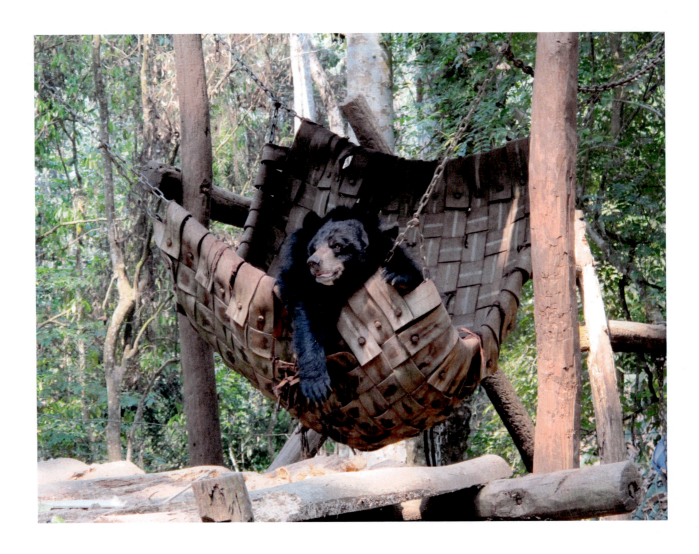

lxiii

Describing Picture Scenes

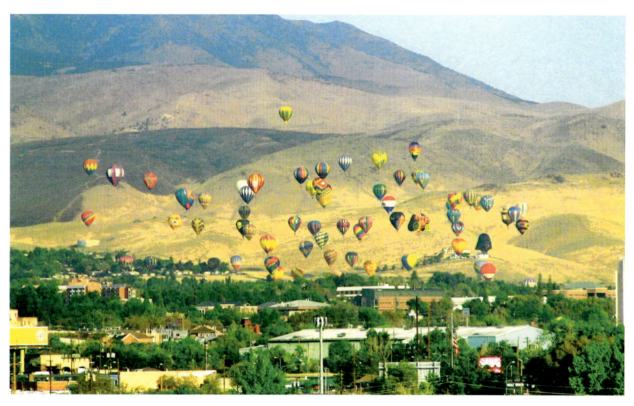

Describing Picture Scenes

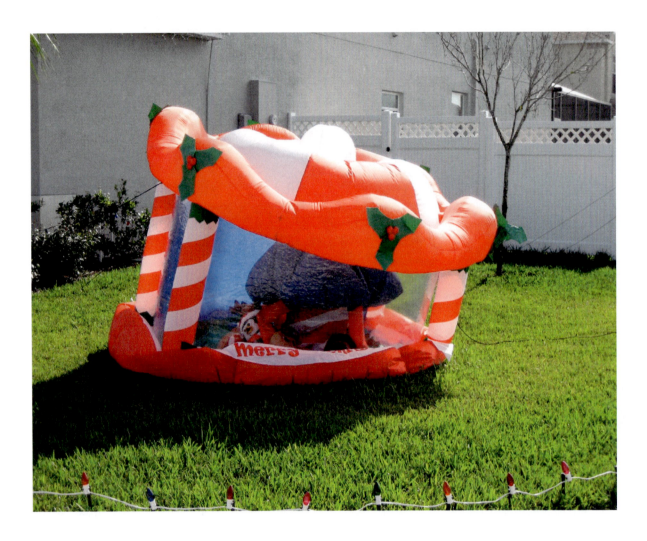

Describing Picture Scenes

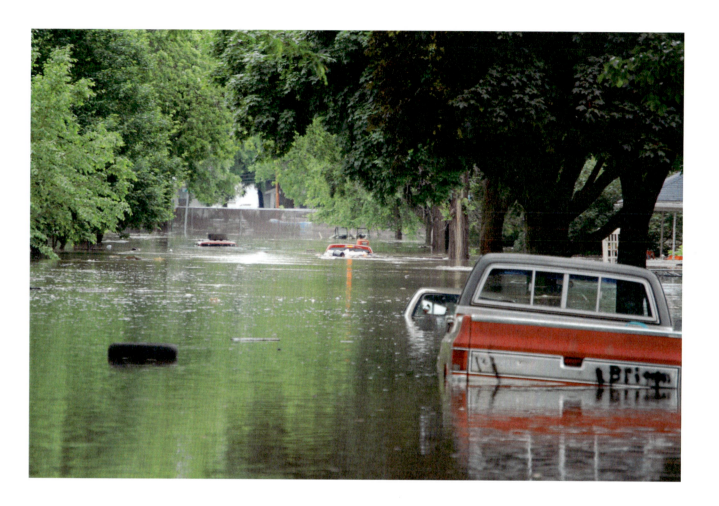

Describing Picture Scenes

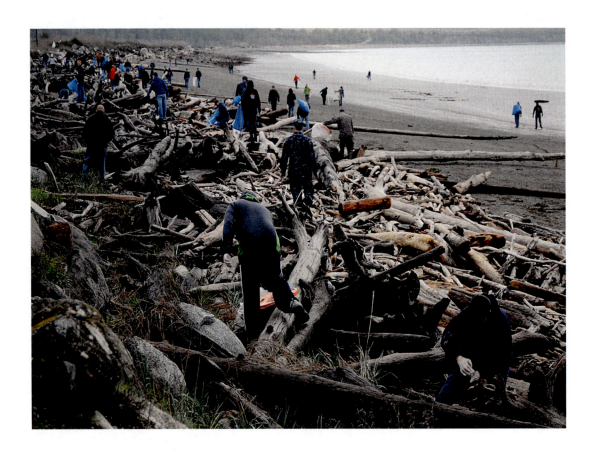

lxvii

Describing Picture Scenes:

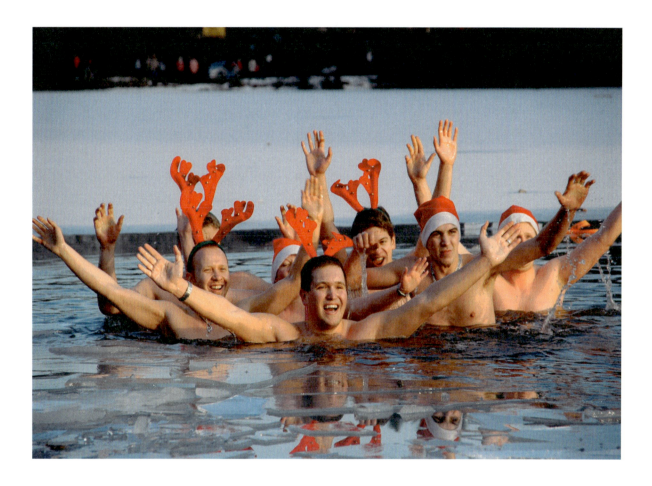

Describing Picture Scenes

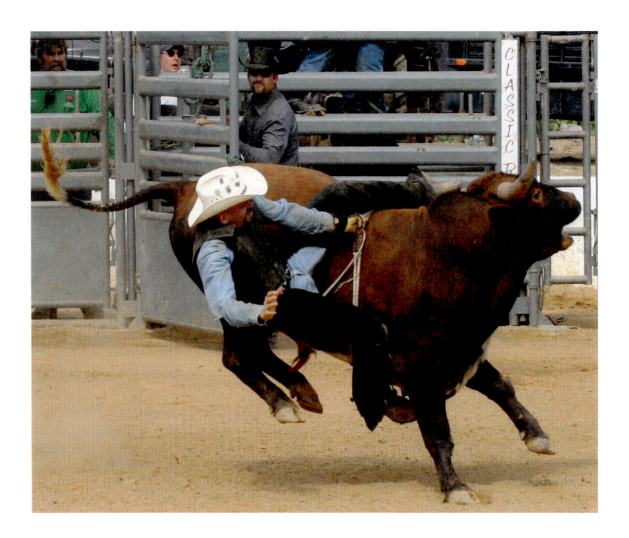

Describing Picture Scenes

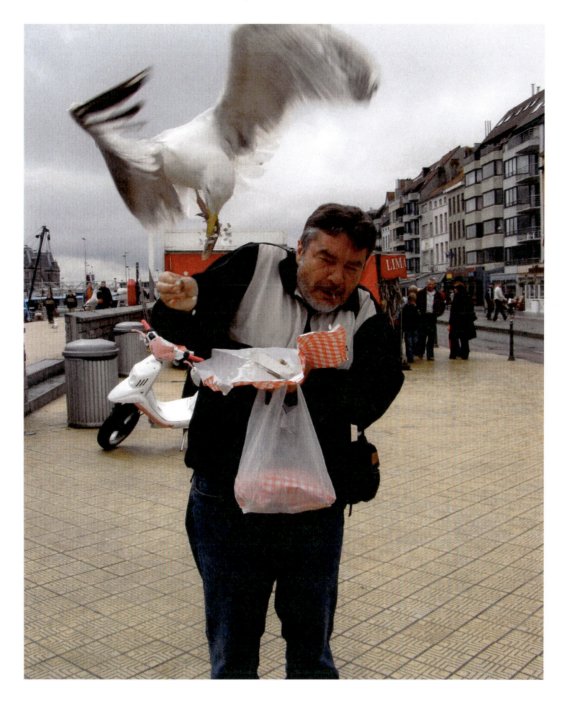

Structured Conversation Sets:

Ask your partner each question. After they answer, have them ask you the same question.

1. How are you today?
2. What is your name?
3. Where are you from?
4. Are you married?
5. Do you have any kids?

Practice the conversation multiple times until your partner is able to answer and ask each question fluently.

1. How are you feeling?
2. Where do you live?
3. Where have your traveled to?
4. What was your favorite place to travel?

1. Do you have any Pets?
2. What kind?
3. What are their names?
4. What do you like to do with them?

Conversation Topics:

Have your partner elaborate as much as possible to answer each question. If you only get a one word answer, continue to ask questions about the topic.

1. Were you ever in a car accident?
2. Did you ever get a speeding or parking ticket?
3. Describe a childhood injury.
4. What was the first date you ever went on?
5. What was your first job?
6. What was the least favorite job you ever had?
7. What was the best job you ever had?
8. What did your father do for a living?
9. What is your mother like?
10. Describe what your family eats and does on Thanksgiving Day.
11. Describe your favorite childhood toy.
12. What sports have you played?
13. What was the best present you ever received?
14. Did you ever break up with somebody?
15. What was the worst trouble you ever got in as a child?
16. Describe your grandparents' house.
17. Where were you when the world trade center was attacked on 9/11/2001?
18. Describe your wedding day.
19. Where did you go for your honeymoon?
20. What was your favorite subject in school?

Conversation Topics:

1. If you could go on vacation anywhere in the world, where would you go and why?
2. What are your thoughts about government regulated gun control?
3. Do you believe that the United States was justified in dropping the Atomic Bomb to end World War II? Why or Why not?
4. In 2012, Colorado and Washington State legalized marijuana for recreational use. What are your thoughts?
5. Tell me about OJ Simpson.
6. Do you believe there is other intelligent life somewhere out there in the universe? Why or why not?
7. What do you think about global warming?
8. What do you think about the death penalty?
9. Dr. Jack Kevorkian spent 8 years in prison for assisting the suicides of 130 terminally ill patients. Do you believe he was a criminal? Why or why not?
10. In 2012, New York City banned sugar drinks over 16 ounces. Do you think the government should restrict the size of soft drinks?
11. Should cigarette smoking be banned?
12. Is torture ever justified?
13. What are your thoughts on the Defense of Marriage Act?
14. What should the United States do about immigration?
15. If you won the lottery, what would you do?

i Source: Jon-Isac Lindberg, CC-BY, via: http://commons.wikimedia.org/wiki/File:White_cup_of_black_coffee.jpg
ii Source: Evan-Amos, CC-BY, via: http://commons.wikimedia.org/wiki/File:Conair-brush.jpg
iii Source: Derick Jensen, CC-BY, via: http://commons.wikimedia.org/wiki/File:Glass-of-water.jpg
iv Source:Charm, CC-BY, via: http://commons.wikimedia.org/wiki/File:Pencil-db.jpg
v Source: Jennifer Dickert, CC-BY, via:
  http://upload.wikimedia.org/wikipedia/commons/7/70/Diamond_ring_photo_by_iLoveButter.jpg
vi Source: Donovan Govan, CC-BY, via http://commons.wikimedia.org/wiki/File:Dessert_Spoon.jpg
vii Source: Jonas Bergsten, CC-BY, via: http://commons.wikimedia.org/wiki/File:Toothbrush_20050716_004.jpg
viii Source: Mk2010, CC-BY, via:http://commons.wikimedia.org/wiki/File:K-
  Swiss_Tubes_Run_100_running_shoe.JPG
ix Source: Evan-Amos, CC-BY, via: http://commons.wikimedia.org/wiki/File:Mach-3-Razor.jpg
x Source: techgizmo, CC-BY, via: http://commons.wikimedia.org/wiki/File:Samsung_Galaxy_S_II_(3).jpg
xi Source: Bangin, CC-BY, via: http://commons.wikimedia.org/wiki/File:Scissor.JPG
xii Source: redjar, CC-BY, via: http://commons.wikimedia.org/wiki/File:Stanley_PowerLock_tape_measure.jpg
xiii Source:Evan-Amos, CC-BY, via: http://commons.wikimedia.org/wiki/File:Lime-Whole-Split.jpg
xiv Source: Chris Barber, CC-BY, via: http://commons.wikimedia.org/wiki/File:Terrier_mixed-breed_dog.jpg
xv Source: Holger Ellgaurd, CC-BY, via: http://commons.wikimedia.org/wiki/File:Flygsmalla_2008.jpg
xvi Source: Cody Escadron Delta, CC-BY, via: http://commons.wikimedia.org/wiki/File:Baseball_ball.jpg
xvii Source: Dvortygirl, CC-BY, via: http://commons.wikimedia.org/wiki/File:Pill_box_with_pills.JPG
xviii Source: Mosborne01, CC-BY, via: http://commons.wikimedia.org/wiki/File:Canon-video-camera.jpg
xix Source: Evan-Amos, CC_BY, via: http://commons.wikimedia.org/wiki/File:Tape-dispenser.jpg
xx Source: Henry Tsing, CC-BY, via: http://commons.wikimedia.org/wiki/File:Fan-shaped_leaf_rake.jpg
xxi Source: PJ, CC-BY, via: http://commons.wikimedia.org/wiki/File:Guitar_1.jpg
xxii Source: Renee Comet, CC-BY, via: http://commons.wikimedia.org/wiki/File:Strawberry_milk_shake.jpg
xxiii Source: Ealdgyth, CC-BY, via: https://commons.wikimedia.org/wiki/File:Felthat.jpg
xxiv Source: Numero 1963, CC-BY, via: http://commons.wikimedia.org/wiki/File:Arrosoir.JPG
xxv Source: Evan-Amos, CC-BY, via: http://commons.wikimedia.org/wiki/File:Cast-Iron-Pan.jpg
xxvi Source: CHG, CC-BY, via: https://commons.wikimedia.org/wiki/File:Mirai_LCD_TV.JPG
xxvii Source: DO'Neil, CC-BY, via: https://commons.wikimedia.org/wiki/File:Showerhead.JPG
xxviii Source: Matthew Bowden, CC-BY, via: https://commons.wikimedia.org/wiki/File:Wasserhahn.jpg
xxix Source: J.Dncsn, CC-BY, via: https://commons.wikimedia.org/wiki/File:White_lamp.JPG
xxx Source: Mets501, CC-BY, via: https://commons.wikimedia.org/wiki/File:Paper_towel.png
xxxi Source: Bangin, CC-BY, via: https://commons.wikimedia.org/wiki/File:Globe.JPG
xxxii Source: Evan Amos, CC-BY, via: http://commons.wikimedia.org/wiki/File:Yorkie-Bar.jpg
xxxiii Source: Peter Kammer, CC-BY, via: http://commons.wikimedia.org/wiki/File:Rollingpin.jpg
xxxiv Source: Evan_Amos, CC-BY, via: http://commons.wikimedia.org/wiki/File:Tool-pliers.jpg
xxxv Source: Badzill, CC-BY, via: http://commons.wikimedia.org/wiki/File:Husqvarna-Rider.jpg
xxxvi Source: Evan-Amos, CC-BY, via: http://upload.wikimedia.org/wikipedia/commons/6/6e/Pepperidge-Farm-
  Nantucket-Cookie.jpg
xxxvii Source: Victorrocha, CC-BY, via: http://commons.wikimedia.org/wiki/File:Half_rim_glasses.JPG
xxxviii Source: Wolfie, CC-BY, via: http://commons.wikimedia.org/wiki/File:Band-Aid_close-up.jpg
xxxix Source: Lars Aronnson, CC-BY, via: http://commons.wikimedia.org/wiki/File:Nsrw1914_2.jpg
xl Source: Evan-Amos, CC-BY, via: http://commons.wikimedia.org/wiki/File:Victor-Mousetrap.jpg
xli Source:: Sam LiskerCC-BY, via: http://en.wikipedia.org/wiki/File:Colt_Model_of_1911_U.S._Army_b.png
xlii Source: Paolo Neo, CC-BY, via:
  http://commons.wikimedia.org/wiki/File:Cigaretet_white_background_stock_photo.jpg
xliii Source: Lotus Head, CC-BY, via: http://commons.wikimedia.org/wiki/File:Credit-cards.jpg
xliv Source: Evan-Amos, CC-BY, via: http://commons.wikimedia.org/wiki/File:Belt-clothing.jpg
xlv Source: Evan-Amos, CC-BY, via: http://commons.wikimedia.org/wiki/File:Kitchen-spatula.jpg

xlvi Source: downtowngirl, CC-BY, via: http://commons.http://upload.wikimedia.org/wikipedia/commons/2/26/Eilat_stone_earrings.jpg

xlvii Source: Iain CC-BY, via: http://commons.wikimedia.org/wiki/File:Fingernail_Clippers.jpg

xlviii Source: Evan-Amos, CC-BY, via: http://commons.wikimedia.org/wiki/File:Pumpkin-Pie-Slice.jpg

xlix Source: Evan-Amos, CC-BY, via: http://commons.wikimedia.org/wiki/File:Handcuffs-Black.jpg

l Source: Evan-Amos, CC-BY, via:http://commons.wikimedia.org/wiki/File:Pink-Frosted-Donut.jpg

li Source: Nevit Dilmen, CC-BY, via: http://commons.wikimedia.org/wiki/File:Swimming_dog_1270213.jpg.

lii Source: Aida, CC-BY, via: http://commons.wikimedia.org/wiki/File:Sz%C3%A9chenyi_Gy%C3%B3gyf%C3%BCrd%C5%91_thermal_spa_in_Budapest_005.JPG

liii Source: Felix Andrews, CC-BY, via: http://commons.wikimedia.org/wiki/File:Mutianyu_tourists.jpg

liv Source: Tuxyso, CC-BY, via: http://commons.wikimedia.org/wiki/File:Mantelaffe-mit-Baby-Zoo-Muenster.jpg

lv Source: Julian Herzog, CC-BY, via: http://commons.wikimedia.org/wiki/File:Lindau_Harbor_Lake_Constance_MS_Schwaben_01.jpg

lvi Source: Ildar Sagdejev CC-BY, via: http://commons.wikimedia.org/wiki/File:2004-05-02_Speed_Limit_3.jpg

lvii Source: Charlesjsharp, CC-BY, via: http://commons.wikimedia.org/wiki/File:Lion_cub_in_rock_cleft.JPG

lviii Source: Ticoles, CC-BY, via: http://commons.wikimedia.org/wiki/File:Scoop_your_poop.jpeg

lix Source: 夢の散歩, CC-BY, via: http://commons.wikimedia.org/wiki/File:%E5%AE%B6%E5%B1%8B%E7%81%AB%E7%81%BDP6014971.jpg

lx Source: U.S. Marine Corps, CC-By via: http://commons.wikimedia.org/wiki/File:USMC-19194.jpg

lxi Source: Sarah Ackerman, CC-BY via: http://commons.wikimedia.org/wiki/File:Pedicure_NYC.jpg

lxii Source: Author's photo, via: Kristin Gurley

lxiii Source: Isderion, CC_BY, via: http://commons.wikimedia.org/wiki/File:Bear_in_Hammock.JPG

lxiv Source: The Conduqtor CC-BY, via: http://commons.wikimedia.org/wiki/File:29th_Annual_Great_Reno_Balloon_Race.JPG

lxv Source: Marcus Quigmire, CC-BY, via:http://commons.wikimedia.org/wiki/File:Dangerous_Carousel_(336393860).jpg

lxvi Source: Don Becker CC-BY, via:http://commons.wikimedia.org/wiki/File:Sunken_cars_on_flooded_street_in_Cedar_Rapids_Iowa.jpg

lxvii Source: Official Navy Page, CC-BY, via: http://commons.wikimedia.org/wiki/File:Flickr_-_Official_U.S._Navy_Imagery_-_Sailors_collect_trash_along_the_beach_at_Costen-Turner_Memorial_Park_to_celebrate_Earth_Day..jpg

lxviii Source: ChBaltes, CC-BY, via:http://commons.wikimedia.org/wiki/File:Ice_swimming_46.jpg

lxix Source: dbking, CC-BY, via: http://commons.wikimedia.org/wiki/File:Don%27t_let_go.jpg

lxx Source: Loki11, CC-BY, via: http://commons.wikimedia.org/wiki/File:Birdsniper.jpg